D1001326

LIFE ETHICS IN
WORLD RELIGIONS

UNIVERSITY OF MANITOBA
STUDIES IN RELIGION

Executive Editor

David G. Creamer

Editorial Board

David G. Creamer
Egil Grislis
Klaus Klostermaier
Dawne C. McCance
Neal Rose
John G. Stackhouse
M. S. Stern

Volume 3

Life Ethics in World Religions

Edited by
Dawne C. McCance

LIFE ETHICS IN WORLD RELIGIONS

Edited by

Dawne C. McCance

Scholars Press
Atlanta, Georgia
1998

LUTHER SEMINARY
LIBRARY
2375 Como Avenue
St. Paul, MN 55108-1447

BJ1188
.L53

LIFE ETHICS IN WORLD RELIGIONS

Edited by

Dawne C. McCance

© 1998
University of Manitoba

Library of Congress Cataloging in Publication Data
Life Ethics in world religions / edited by Dawne McCance.
    p.   cm. — (University of Manitoba studies in religion ; v. 3)
    Includes bibliographical references and index.
    ISBN 0-7885-0452-5 (pbk. : alk. paper)
    1. Religious ethics. 2. Bioethics—Religious aspects.
I. McCance, Dawne, 1944– . II. Series.
BJ1188.L54   1998
291.5'697—dc21   98-16689

Printed in the United States
on acid-free paper

ALDO-29601

Contents

Introduction

I. Traditional Perspectives

II. Contemporary Challenges

PREFACE

The purpose of the *University of Manitoba Studies in Religion* is to publish work that reflects the study of religion in a public university. The diversity of religious traditions discussed in the following essays, as well as the disciplinary diversity of the contributors, are representative of the study of religion at public universities in North America.

The inaugural volume in this monograph series (*Goddesses in Religions and Modern Debate*, 1990), based on a 1988 colloquium series organized by the University of Manitoba's Department of Religion, embodies substantial discussions of particular goddess traditions and controversial questions in current literature on "the divine feminine."

On the occasion of the twentieth anniversary of the Department of Religion at the University of Manitoba, thirty scholars from across Canada and around the world gathered for a conference—"Religious Studies: Directions for the Next Two Decades." The papers presented, which reflected on the past of the discipline, its present status, and future possibilities, form the content of the second volume in the series, *Religious Studies: Issues, Prospects and Proposals* (1991).

A great deal of planning and effort has gone into this third volume of the series. The scholarly efforts of the contributors will be obvious to the reader. Not so obvious to those who have not attempted to massage a work through the editing and production stages is the time-consuming labor involved in preparing a "camera ready" manuscript for printing. Dawne McCance and I have renewed appreciation for the intricacies of "desk top publishing." Even with the help of sophisticated computer technology and *The Chicago Manual of Style* the process has been lengthy. Thanks are due to Gladys Broesky of the Jesuit Centre at St. Paul's College, the University of Manitoba, for her work in formatting and correcting the manuscript at its various stages, and to Michael Caligiuri for his help with the Index. I don't think we would ever have finished the project without the help of a Scholars Press "Editor's Workshop," which I attended in September of 1997. Thanks to Harry Gilmer, Denis Ford and the entire staff of Scholars Press for their interest in and encouragement of this project.

Winnipeg   David G. Creamer
March, 1998   Executive Editor

INTRODUCTION

Life Ethics in World Religions:
What this Book is About

Dawne C. McCance

Let's begin with *life ethics*. Since deciding on the title of this book, I have had
several inquiries as to the meaning of the term *life ethics*. We are more familiar
with *bioethics*, the name of a whole new field of ethical inquiry that has flourished
over the past three decades. Bioethics is often dated to the late 1960's and the
founding of the Hastings Center in New York. Along with other centers that
opened shortly thereafter (such as the Kennedy Institute of Ethics in Washington,
DC, and the Center for Bioethics in Montréal), the Hastings Center initiated a
wave of interdisciplinary research and consultation, course offerings, and publications in moral and ethical issues associated with theoretical and technological
developments in the biological and biomedical fields. Bioethics rose quickly to
prominence as a public discourse, as a profession, and as a multi-faceted area of
academic study, and in every case, it encouraged ethical reflection on such issues
as prenatal diagnosis, abortion, *in vitro* fertilization, eugenics, gene therapy, DNA
recombination research, health resource allocation, use of life-sustaining tech-
nologies, organ transplantation, and euthanasia. Many bioethical anthologies and
collections of essays appeared, but perhaps not surprisingly, these were given for
the most part to Western philosophical, primarily Anglo-American, ethical perspectives. A lesser number of theological contributions, most of them Christian,
made up the religious ethics component of these early bioethics collections.

If this book were a reader in bioethics, its appearance would thus be timely.
For we need more studies that bring religious ethics to bear on the so-called
bioethical issues with which we are struggling today. Too often, bioethics has
been reduced to the application of an historically-recent and culturally-specific
rights-based paradigm, without regard for the ethical diversity that must needs be
respected in a post-colonial world. This book, we might say, redresses the problem
in that it discusses some bioethical issues—among them wartime killing, suicide,
contraception, reproduction and ecology—from different religious ethics

perspectives. Diversity is maintained: the essays collected here represent multi-cultural points of view.

What the essays have in common is an interest in the ethics of life. The word "bioethics" means literally this, "ethics of life," and yet the essays assembled here conceive of life ethics as, necessarily, encompassing more than analysis of biomedical problems and possibilities. The term *life ethics* is retained in the book title to allow for this wider scope. The essays extend the range of bioethics to a number of the world's religious traditions and thus to some very different interpretations of life, and of ethics, than prevail in the contemporary West. The book is as much about these differences in interpretation of life and of ethical living as it is about the resolution of this or that issue. Increased awareness of these differences could, radically, open new options for the bioethical movement.

The idea that new perspectives might derive from very old systems of ethics suggests another thread that ties these very different essays together: they represent the on-going, living, research of ten Canadian scholars currently working, in one way or another, in traditional ethical systems. Their research demonstrates that ethical traditions, even ancient ones, are perpetually being re-lived. *Life Ethics in World Religions* aims to bring this research-in-process into the classroom setting. While it should appeal to student and scholar alike, the book is designed as a textbook for undergraduate religious studies and bioethics courses. This means that although the essays are selective studies, they are written so as to provide the basis for a larger investigation of the ethical traditions in question. For example, David Creamer's essay in Chapter Seven provides an analysis of Bernard Lonergan's reinterpretation of the Roman Catholic natural law ethical tradition, particularly as it applies to the question of contraception. The essay lends itself to a teaching situation in which discussion could effectively move to Roman Catholic natural law ethics in general, as well as to its historical application to other issues such as suicide and abortion, and to the contemporary re-examination of natural law ethics in the context of such questions as homosexuality and *in vitro* fertilization. The Roman Catholic natural law approach could be compared to other ways of doing Christian ethics, and so on: the essays are offered as points of departure for classroom discussion.

Generally, the first eight essays in the collection are arranged in chrono-logical order, and are studies centered in specific religious traditions. The collection opens with Katharine Bitney's attempt to articulate the life ethics framework—the world-view foundation, ethical principles, and conduct appli-cations—implicit in Goddess religion. We cannot return to prehistory, Bitney points out in "Ethics and the Goddess," but we can, through the Goddess, re-imagine contemporary life ethics. The classroom might be a place to start: so

Laara Fitznor suggests in the second essay in this volume, "The Circle of Life: Affirming Aboriginal Philosophies in Everyday Living." These Aboriginal philosophies are all-but-absent from available religious ethics and bioethics anthologies, and yet, as Fitznor explains, the philosophies are rooted in ways of looking at the world (at the circle of life) that, especially today, need to be understood and practiced.

The question of how life ethics teachings are, in fact, practiced in life, is at the heart of the following three essays. Eva Neumaier's "Buddhists within the Moral Space of Non-Duality" provides a good basis for classroom discussion of the Buddhist tradition and its Theravada and Mahayana ethical systems, with their emphasis on non-injury, equanimity and compassion. The essay also considers the lives of some exemplary, ancient and contemporary, Buddhists, asking whether their actual behavior can be said to accord with the ethical norms that they embraced. In Chapter Four, "The Life-Ethics of the Bhagavadgītā as Interpreted by Rāmānuja," Klaus Klostermaier turns to the life ethics of another ancient tradition, Hinduism, as presented in the Bhagavadgītā. Reading the Gītā along with Rāmānuja, Klostermaier finds in it a Hindu "life ethics" that is, again, very different from the recent Western model, particularly as concerns the understanding of life as a whole. In practice, this ethics does not rule out the taking of life or the waging of war, but it does consider these to be religious and moral, rather than legal or political questions; a distinction that Klostermaier underlines. Albert Welter's "Life, Death and Enlightenment: Buddhist Ethics in a Chinese Context," returns to Buddhist ethical teachings as understood and practiced in a Chinese context. The essay examines the life of an individual practitioner, Yung-ming Yen-shou (904–975), a military official who, on converting to Buddhism, became increasingly unable to live out his military role. Moved by the Buddhist ideal of compassion, Yen-shou went so far as to appropriate funds under his command to buy living creatures and set them free. The essay explores Yen-shou's defense of terminating one's life as well as his integration of Confucian ethics into a Buddhist framework.

Chapters Six, Seven and Eight center in the Biblical traditions of Judaism, Christianity and Islam, and in the complex question of adapting traditional ethics to the present-day world. In "Revisioning Judaism: Mordecai Kaplan's Ethics of Immanence," Neal Rose interprets Judaism as an ethics of ritual that is based in the tradition's *lauch*, its Sacred Calendar. The essay introduces students to the *halachah,* the traditional, Rabbinic, way of living the *lauch*, and at the same time it presents Kaplan's understanding of the *lauch* as a major modern attempt to reconstitute the Jewish ethical tradition. Another attempt at reconstructing traditional ethics is taken up by David Creamer in "Bernard J. F. Lonergan:

Existential Ethics." For Lonergan, as for Kaplan, modern historical and scientific knowledges make necessary a rethinking of traditional ethics. Creamer provides an accessible introduction to Lonergan's method of deriving an existential ethics from the knowing process, always connecting this ethics to responsible decision-making about the use of artificial contraception. In Chapter Eight, the focus shifts to gender issues. Sheila McDonough's "Gender Hierarchy and Ethics in Islamic Thought" both introduces readers to Muslim ethics and critically analyzes the tradition's assumptions concerning gender hierarchy in the context of marriage and family life, separation of the sexes and veiling of the woman. Issues of gender hierarchy are vigorously debated among Muslims in the twentieth century, McDonough points out: this tradition, too, is going through the process of adaptation.

The final section of the book continues, and focuses, the question of contemporary challenges to traditional religious life ethics. Morny Joy's "Feminist Scholarship: the Challenge to Ethics" undertakes a three-part thematic analysis of the last twenty years of feminist ethics, highlighting some of the major trends that have appeared and drawing out their relevance for religious ethics. The essay provides students with a provocative analysis of a range of source material and with a thoughtful introduction to the many issues that feminism brings to religious ethics. Harold Coward's "Are There Religious Responses to Global Ethical Issues?" contends that today's challenges of over population, excess consumption of the world's resources and pollution of earth, air and water are new ethical problems that call for new responses from traditional ethics. Coward's essay outlines some work that he has done in exploring the identity of the traditional ethical agent. In traditional cultures, he says, ethical agents are given a collective identity, a "We-Self," that is quite distinct from the autonomous individual "I-Self" of Western liberal ethics. The distinction makes a conceptual and practical difference, as Coward's case-studies explain. His essay brings the book to a fitting close, for it suggests that awareness of the differences brought by the "We-Self" ideal could, as I mention above, open new options for the contemporary life ethics movement.

PART I

TRADITIONAL PERSPECTIVES

Chapter 1

Ethics and the Goddess

Katharine Bitney

There is a Neo-pagan joke that made the rounds a few years ago: "The Goddess is back, and boy is She mad." A variation of the joke went like this: "God is back, and boy is She mad." The variation was meant as a direct rebuttal to Nietzsche's "God is dead" theory. Yet it was more. It spoke to the endurance of belief in divinity, certainly: Nietzsche can no more kill God than can a million skeptics and atheists. But God changes, or rather, human perceptions, imaginative constructions and experiences of God change. They always have. Perhaps Nietzsche was right in a sense: God as we have known It is dead, or dying, or mutating, or being replaced. The joke, however, does more than refute the notion that humans no longer need or believe in God (they do, it seems, more than ever); it changes God's gender (back) from male to female, definitely and firmly.

Let's unpack both these versions of the joke. In the second version, the surprise is that God has changed gender from male to female. This is meant to shock a world which simply assumes a male identity to the Ultimate, that "Lord" is the nth degree of Being, creativity and authority, that "He" is the automatic ascription of gender when speaking of divinity. "And boy is She mad" only hints that either God has changed gender (again?) or that She was female all along and nobody noticed, or that true divinity has been shoved aside or sleeping for all the millennia of patriarchy.

In the first version, the gender of God reverts to its original status: female. "The Goddess is back." It is as though the male God was an aberration, or as though divine gender has been misread, or as though the female divine had been pushed aside, or had stepped aside to let Her "son(s)" have a go at world management. Certainly it speaks to an understanding, an assumption, that *originally*, God was female (this is corroborated now by the archaeological record). The "coming back" of the Goddess is different from the "coming back" of God: for Him, it is recognition that He never really went away. But for Her, it is a much longer return, from the depths of history and prehistory, of collective unconscious, from human genetic memory. It is as though She were being awakened or She had seen enough of what happens when She lets the boys manage things, and is returning to step in and set things right. If She is back, where has she been? And what is She so mad about?

I would like to address both these questions by way of considering the issues raised in the theme of this essay: Ethics and the Goddess. I would like to consider the connections between ethics, justice and the female divine as we have it in mythology and common parlance (Justice as a female figure, for example), and read back in time to eras when the female divine still had devotional, judicial and retributive power. I would like to consider the origins of such ascriptions in greater antiquity, reading back to earliest theological structures, descending from the Neo-, Meso- and Paleolithic by reading archaeological and anthropological data. For us in the West, the Goddess is back from those times and from under the suppression of patriarchy with the contemporary rise of Neo-paganism, the revival of Witchcraft and the development of feminist Goddess spirituality. Her coming back implies more than simple divine gender change. It signals a different theology which in turn proposes a different source and reading of ethics.

Who or what is the Goddess? "The Goddess is multi-faceted, ever-changing —nature and nature's transformations," writes Luhrmann (Luhrmann, *Persuasions of Witch's Craft*, 46). From Geoffrey Ashe: "The Goddess was and is the Great Mother, Earth rather than sky, the life bestower, the creative energy, the giver of birth and rebirth, within nature" (Ashe, *Dawn Behind the Dawn*, 11). And from Starhawk: "The Goddess . . . *is* reality, the manifest deity, omnipresent in all of life, in each of us. The Goddess is not separate from the world—She *is* the world, and all things in it . . ." (Starhawk, *The Spiral Dance*, 22).

These are modern writers, presenting us with a reading of the female divine as Nature itself: as energy and mind together, creating and destroying in order to create again; as bestower, taker and regenerator of life. The drama of birth, death and rebirth does not take place outside the Goddess but within Her: the universe is seen and experienced as the divine body itself. As "parts" of a whole body, the many facets and factors of nature do not exist apart from each other, but as interconnected strands of the whole: all depends on all. For Western minds, this categorizing of the divine as immanent is a radical departure from the theologies of divine transcendence we have become accustomed to. It is in this way, in terms of immanence rather than transcendence, that Goddess is most different from God.

God is a somewhat distant ruler. But, as Starhawk points out, "The Goddess does not rule the world—She is the world" (*The Spiral Dance*, 23)—the world, the life force, creativity, risk. As to her body the Universe, it has a tendency to exist. We are not externalized, apart from the divine, but part of it. What alienates us from the divine is hubris: we imagine not only that we are not part of the divine, but the divine is apart from us. This separation from divine nature may give the appearance of divine order, but it does not reflect intuited reality. In Goddess theology, divine order comes from within nature/goddess. In God theology, it is imposed from outside.

If the Goddess is "back," how did She get "lost" in the first place? When and where did She disappear from the Western pantheon (for disappear She did, since She was most certainly there from the beginning)? A current version of the history of the divine in the West goes something like this: the earliest images we have of the divine, dating from the Paleolithic, are female. This fact is confirmed and reconfirmed by the archaeological record. Images of the Great Mother insist on Her supremacy, Her abundance, Her life-giving attributes, Her immanence in nature and Her authority in the giving and taking of life.

As human life transformed from hunter/gatherer societies to agricultural settlements, the role of the Goddess as source of fertility intensified, and agriculture brought with it a new source of responsibility and guilt: tearing up the body of the Mother. Some groups of people, however, became pastoralists and domesticated animals which they moved from place to place. It is in the story of these people that we find the first inklings of a supreme male God supplanting the Goddess, and the first inklings of patriarchy, male domination. About 5000 years ago, these newly patriarchal people began to swoop down on the agricultural people and to impose both their theology and their social order. The Goddess began to fragment and was gradually demoted to wife, sister, daughter. Eventually, she was eliminated altogether in favor of one supreme transcendent male deity. This is where we find ourselves today. However, there have always been small pockets of old believers who have carried the old ways down through time despite persecution, until the present day. "The Goddess is back," because her believers are "back." But perhaps more importantly, She is back because She is needed, because world conditions (pollution, world population explosion, gender imbalance, etc.) require a return to a theology of immanence in order to restore balance and vitality to the *whole* of planet earth. Survival of the entire biosphere is at stake, not just the survival of humans.

There was a time when natural law, divine law and human (ethical) law were one and the same, when one was not disconnected from the other, when the exercise of power in one area touched on the others. I would like to use the image of the Egyptian Goddess Maat to symbolize this connection. Of her, Merlin Stone writes that she is "the manifestation of truth, justice, moral law and cosmic balance" (Stone, *Ancient Mirrors of Womanhood*, 260). The word "maat" can mean balance, harmony, law, justice, truth, and refers to both Nature and human behavior. Her symbols are a feather and the scales, indicating that balance and natural law have long been connected. According to Baring and Cashford, Maat is "the goddess through whom the fundamental laws of the universe became visible. She embodies truth, right order, lawfulness and justice" (Baring and Cashford, *The Myth of the Goddess*, 261). "Social order was then a reflection of divine order" (261). Maat is, then, "an image of cosmic order—archetypal harmony or universal law—which human social order, and, in Egypt, even the principles of musical harmony derive from and reflect" (263). For, "'in the beginning' it was an inherently feminine conception expressing the spiritual order of the whole and the law of incarnation governing the principles whereby unity became manifest as diversity" (263). An Egyptian prayer reveals the inter-connection of all things in Maat, harmony:

> Your right eye is Maat, your left eye is Maat
> your flesh, your members are Maat
> your food is Maat, your drink is Maat
> the breaths of your nose are Maat
> you exist because Maat exists
> and she exists because you exist.

How far back then, might this conception of spiritual order and incarnation as "inherently feminine" go? Certainly we know that images of the Goddess are associated with law and justice in Sumerian, Egyptian and Greek culture: Inanna as lawgiver, Demeter as lawgiver, Gaia (Mother Earth) as lawgiver, female figures such as the Furies, Nemesis and Dike are associated with law, fate and retribution. If Goddess is lawgiver, then law originates in the nature of Her being and Her being is nature itself. The original oracle of truth at Delphi was Gaia, the Mother Earth, nature. And we know that the presence, even the supremacy, of the Goddess can be extrapolated back to the Paleolithic, before agriculture, to the dawn of human culture.

Since the order of the Goddess reaches back so far, let's consider Her ethics, Her justice as emanating from survival. We know from archaeological evidence that life and time were seen and experienced as circular, cyclical. The earliest Neanderthal burials reveal that rebirth of some kind was anticipated by the use of red ochre and pollen in graves. This habit of burying with ochre, pollen, sometimes with vulva-shaped cowrie shells, continued well into the later Stone

Ages among modern humans, suggesting that rebirth was assumed to be as natural as the return of birds or plants in spring. A circular sense of time encloses life within a biosphere of returning and recycling, and this also means spirit. The idea of *karma*, spiritual growth through many lives working out positive and negative effects, originates in this cyclical vision of life: spirit and matter are not separate, but flow in and out of each other, affect each other. "Sin," or unethical behavior, pollutes the earth itself, alters the conditions of the world around us.

For the earliest people, learning to survive by trial and error, would have necessitated keen observation of natural cycles and natural occurrences such as death producing new life, the interdependence of plants and animals, and the necessity for humans to live within the means of a given ecosystem, never taking more than it could provide: there is no shortage of cautionary tales about hunters taking more than they needed, and causing starvation or the disappearance of prey species. Greed therefore creates an ethical dilemma because it creates a survival dilemma. Respect for all (non-human) life becomes an ethical issue. The prey is understood to give itself to the hunter, thus the prey animal becomes a teacher in the ethics of self-sacrifice. Some theriomorphic deities are pictured as prey animals, for example the Celtic god Cernunnos as a stag, to remind people that all food comes from the divine body. If the Goddess as life-giver is immanent in all things, then we are partaking of the divine body itself. (Theophagy begins in a theology of immanence!)

Likewise, in order to survive, groups require rules to maximize cooperation, and a reproductive ethics that will ensure a stable and manageable population inhabiting an area. The health and vigor of a population demands rigorous marriage rules—and so on. So one might say that in the ancient universe of the Goddess, survival of humans rests in the context of the survival of, and in relation to, each other, and all other species. Such ethics may be said to be grounded in survival and the collective. The more complex the life system, the more complex the ethics.

"Goddess" ethics are rooted in the embodied divine: so, the value of bodiliness rises when the foundation of bodiliness is the divine itself: in Goddess theology, bodiliness is an aspect of divine nature. It is perhaps in this area that Goddess most radically differs from God. Goddess theology is pantheistic. This is a problematic theology for the Western mind: first because we are accustomed to considering divinity to be pure spirit, too "high" or too "divine" to be body (thus automatically lowering the value of matter); and because "all" includes ourselves—we are part of the divine—and this implies that "evil" is potential within the divine.

Certainly, the doing of evil is a risk the divine/nature takes when offering consciousness and choice as an evolutionary probability to a species. As that particular species, we humans learn by trial and error what is good and what is evil, and, when we know the difference, we know what God knows. Writers of the Bible recognized that knowledge of good and evil is a risky business, and is divine knowledge. Where a modern Goddess worshiper would differ from the writers of Genesis is in the right of humans to divine knowledge: a patriarchal reading would be "no, we have no right to it because we are creatures of the divine"; a Goddess-oriented reading would be "yes, because we are part of the divine, it is our knowledge of ourselves: it is a way for the divine to know itself, or, it is a way for nature to experience its own manifold possibilities."

But how do we distinguish between good and evil? How do we decide which is which? From the "Goddess" point of view, we begin by assuming sacrality, divinity in everything, including ourselves. What is "evil" may be deemed that which mitigates against survival, against life, does deliberate harm —not only interspecially, but intraspecially. It is important to differentiate here between natural disasters and functions such as floods, droughts and so on, which deliver "evil" results, and deliberate conscious evil such as war, rape, murder and ecological devastation. The former is merely the movement of nature toward internal balance; no harm is intended; it is just the cosmos in a condition of self-creation. The latter, however, is predicated on human choice of action. Deliberate harm is intended. This harm is inflicted in a mode of what Starhawk, Eisler and others refer to as "power-over." We might say that unethical behavior occurs as a misuse of power, the exercise of power over others, over our own species, and over the rest of nature, to the extent that that is possible. The difference between natural events which do harm and human events which do harm is, essentially, intent. Where the intent of an exercise in power is harm, we might say evil has been done, and that natural ethics have been breached. The Wiccan ethical law, "Harm None," derives from this understanding, and applies to any exercise of power and will in the life world. Any choice of action, by individual or group resonates throughout the entire web of life, the universe itself.

If we view human ethics as rooted in survival, how does the misuse of power endanger survival? Obviously, it can threaten or inflict harm on individuals or groups: murder or war negate individual and collective survival, for example. Or, environmental devastation can threaten the survival of entire populations, entire ecosystems, even the survival of individual species. At what point did humans lose their sense of ethics based on survival as a species within a whole system, and push through to an ethic based on human (or individual) supremacy?

When did cosmic (and social/ethical) order, what I have symbolized as Maat, change from balance to conquest?

Writers like Baring and Cashford, Riane Eisler, Starhawk and others support the theory of the pastoral invaders: Aryans from the Northeast, and Semites from the south, entering and sacking the "peaceful Goddess worshiping" agricultural people of the middle-east and southern Europe, bringing with them their thunderous sky gods: "Both invading peoples introduced the idea of an opposition between the powers of light and darkness, imposing this polarity on the older view in which the whole contained both light and darkness in an ever-changing relationship" (Baring and Cashford, *The Myth of the Goddess*, 157). Baring and Cashford argue that "The belief in the absolute separation between humanity and the deity is contrary to the Neolithic agriculturalist's vision" (157), which sees "the goddess as immanent in all life" (157). This encounter left us with "two 'historical souls'" (158), an "ethos of conquest" (158) overlaid on an ethos of natural harmony. They write:

> The moral order of the goddess culture . . . was based on the principle of the relationship of the manifest to the unmanifest, where the manifest was the epiphany . . . of the unmanifest. . . . The moral order of the god culture . . . was based on the paradigm of opposition and conquest: a view of life, and particularly of nature, as something 'other' to be conquered. The manifest world was seen as intrinsically separate from the unmanifest world, which was now placed outside or beyond nature in the realm of the transcendent gods. (Baring and Cashford, *The Myth of the Goddess*, 158)

It begs the question of how an ethos of conquest, dualisms and othering may be viewed in terms of survival, if survival is our chosen ground of ethics. If survival is imagined to be in spite of, or in opposition to, nature, then such an ethos might be viewed as survival-based, but over against, and not in harmony with, the rest of the natural world. Humans in this ethos "other" themselves from the larger natural world, and from other groups of humans. Even survival after death changes in this ethos: "death came to be regarded as the absolute end and opposite of life . . . Darkness was now associated with what was *not* light or life, rather than, as in the lunar mythology, with the disappearance of manifestation and the place from which new life was born. Death became something final, terrifying, remorseless, and without the promise of rebirth" (Baring & Cashford, 159). Death becomes an enemy of life, in this world view, rather than an aspect of it: death, too, is "other." The ethical implications and results of this perspective we live with even today, including such remedies to death as overpopulation and the attendant oppression of women, and such remedies to overpopulation as exploitation and devastation of the earth, and war.

"The Goddess is back, and boy is She mad." Why is the Goddess back? It's not like She has always been gone from everywhere in the world. There are and always have been places where She never left, or if She left, She returned: India, for example, or some parts of Africa; among "primitive" people living close to the edge in all parts of the world, the Goddess has always been a presence. The Kogi of South America, for instance, have always recognized the creator as female, Aluna, whose divine imagination contemplated the workings of every marvelous facet of nature.

Here in the West, She has had much further to come: from the depths of antiquity, from under the shadow of the self-proclaimed supreme single male deity. And even here She has lurked in the shadows of remnant paganism, as public symbol (the figure of Justice with her scales and sword comes to mind) and, sanitized, in the folds of the Christian cloak, as the Virgin Mary. Even here we have never stopped referring to nature and the earth as Mother.

Let's return to the idea of Nature (Goddess) as lawgiver (Gaia, Demeter, Inanna, for example). It tells us that ethics are, as it were, woven into the fabric of nature itself, imprinted in genetic material. Law (as an expression of an ethos) does not come from outside nature in this world view. Law does not fall from the heavens and impose itself on the world; it is not transcendent of nature in the world of the Goddess. Law arises from the Goddess Herself. And yet, from within our outmoded ethos, we speak of, indeed insist upon, the laws of nature in the study of science, but not in philosophy, not in ethics, not in the study of human law. Why not? In the world of Maat, they are all the same thing.

"The Goddess is back . . ." Why? How did she get back through the layers and layers of linearity and absolutism and teleology and the patriarchal fantasy of "progress"? Why is the Old Religion being renewed, with its theology of immanence and its return to the Goddess? In part, one suspects, because the current structures, and the current ethos, are no longer answering or speaking to the deepest issues of survival, not only of the human species, but of the whole planet. The current distribution (and exercise) of power is endangering all life. The patriarchal desperation to impose "order" on (what is interpreted as chaotic) life on earth is losing its ability to manage the problems arising out of its own inequity, its own iniquity, and its own terror and mistrust of natural chaos. Dualizing, compartmentalizing and controlling, hallmarks of patriarchy, create more fires than they are able to put out.

At the core of this problem is the imposition of male power over females, reflected in the mythological record as the demotion of the Goddess to wife, daughter, consort: roughly translatable as male (human) power over nature and her representative, woman; making her manageable, rather than, as in the old way, working as a partner with her. From the standpoint of Goddess ethics, this imposition of power-over (male over female) constitutes a condition of harm, which sets in motion, and perpetuates, a chain of harmful effects: an imbalance (of power) which sets off a reaction of imbalances throughout nature. If we look at nature from the point of view of particle physics, we see not so much objects as a state or condition of energy always in flux, motion and reaction. If one particle is changed, the whole field of energy from end to end of the universe changes. Likewise in the "human-sized world," a negative or harmful event initiated some-where in the field, or web, of life, or body of the Goddess, alters and affects all other events in the universe. In Goddess ethics, one is responsible to the entire universe when exercising the powers inherent in choice of action.

If we view the change in consciousness from cyclical to linear, from Goddess to God, as occurring within nature, then we can say that the whole of nature has altered from within its own body: the divine risk of giving con-sciousness to a single species has created an imbalance within the universe, the divine body. Perhaps we can look at the return of the Goddess as a natural necessity for the recalibration of natural balance: Maat's scales, if you like, weighing together cosmos and human ethics: heart and feather.

But the universe is dynamic, not static, and the Goddess (nature) is continually creating new species. To do this, old species have to disappear. Imbalance is necessary for the departure of old species and the creation of new ones: for example, the demise of the dinosaurs was essential for the rise of mammalian, avian and other species. This speaks to an inexorable law of nature: things have to die so new things can live. One could argue that the imbalances created by the pushing aside of the Goddess and imposition of (male human/divine) rule are a necessary part of nature in flux and creativity. Perhaps. But one might also argue that the degree to which this imbalance has been pushed is endangering too much of terrestrial life: we are fouling our own nest.

The imposition of male/transcendent divine rule, and the exclusion of the immanent female divine, have altered our reading of cosmic law as well as human ethics: primarily, in the area of disconnection, because a transcendent divine disconnects humans from the divine, from the rest of nature, and from each other. We no longer recognize the "other" as self. By disconnecting from the divine we change our construction of responsibility: our allegiance is not to this world, but to the next, to a transcendent divinity who demands obedience to himself (there is a certain desperation in such a divinity, as we can read in the Old Testament). We are now caretakers of God's garden, or exploiters of God's gifts, depending on our theology. Our survival depends on God's grace, not on our own actions and behavior toward the rest of the world. Our disconnection from nature, and from each other, creates the false impression that there is "other," and allows for just such an ethos as the justification of conquest to arise and to perpetuate itself, like an insidious strand of moral DNA that has insinuated itself into our consciousness, a parasite that has made itself at home in the body of the Goddess and transformed Her into a rapacious Him. No wonder She's so mad!

It's no accident that the return of the Goddess is driven by women, by feminists, who see in the Goddess, not only themselves, female, but a return to, or reimagining of, the original ethical structure of immanence, cyclicity, bodiliness and interconnection, and natural justice through karmic cycles. Central to this restructuring of ethics is the recalibration of the male–female relationship, in terms of power-sharing and valuing.

In her book, *The Chalice and the Blade*, Riane Eisler identifies two types of societies: dominator and partnership. At the core of domination or partnership in cultures is the female–male relationship: where males dominate females, societies "have generally hierarchic and authoritarian social structure and a high degree of social violence, particularly warfare" (Eisler, *The Chalice and the Blade*, xix); where the genders are more or completely equal (partnership), "such 'partnership model' societies tend to be not only much more peaceful but also much less hierarchic and authoritarian" (xix). Indeed, again and again writers note that gender equality and peacefulness seem to go hand in hand, socially and politically. The Goddess–worshiping culture of old Crete is often pointed to as a model of the ideal partnership society. Eisler argues that transcending "the conventional polarities between right and left, capitalism and communism, religion and secularism, and even masculanism and feminism" (xix–xx), moves societies toward partnership. The dualisms (male–female, spirit–matter, dark–light, life–death and so on, one always privileged over the other) constructed by the early patriarchal societies, and which remain with us even today, perpetuate dominator–model social and political structures and behaviors. As we have seen, these dualities and constructs are symbolized and legitimized theologically by the distant transcendent (male) deity. It is a lopsided universe presided over by a fearful and rather lonely deity, a false and artificial ethos imposed upon, rather than arising out of, the natural world. Feminist thinkers of both genders would (and do) argue that for the sake of a human evolutionary future, and the future of this planet, a change in ethics and theology, toward something like Eisler's "partnership model" is essential. And many of them would argue that a return to, or *of*, the Goddess, is central to this project.

For one thing, the Goddess:

> is a deity who bestows respect and admiration upon the spheres women have traditionally occupied. She is an invitation to human women to proudly claim a special female identification with nature and the body, with sexuality and childbirth, . . . Her femaleness is not solely a matter of biological sex but an identification with things denigrated as feminine and an opposition to ideals uplifted as manly. (Eller, *Living in the Lap of the Goddess*, 135)

We might identify the ethos of conquest with its sky gods as promoting "ideals uplifted as manly." Eller points out that "The nexus of values gathered under the goddess's skirts include the sanctity of nature, the earth and the moon, the life of the body, and sexuality" (135). In "Goddess" (immanentist) terms, bodiliness itself is an aspect of, rather than just something constructed by, the divine; therefore, it is not something to transcend but to value and celebrate. Here, the body is valued as an occasion of spirituality. In this (Goddess) ethos, a valued body might be imagined as a site and/or instrument of worship and ethical behavior. It is not used, nor does it use itself, as a weapon. It is not raped nor does it rape. It does not nor is it murder(ed). It is not "other," nor fallen. It is sacred.

"Nothing is lost in the Goddess" (Eller, 139). Likewise, nothing is missing from the Goddess, including the response and forces of natural justice, the rise and fall of the cycles of creation, destruction and re-creation. If She is all, then She contains all possibility, including the possibility for expressing the negative. Yet She rights herself when the scales tip too far away from the survival of Her members, when cosmic harmony and human justice veer too far away from each other, as they have during this patriarchal (dominator) age. That's why She's back. And that's why She's so mad.

Can we go back to that distant, (perhaps too idealized) Goddess world? Of course not, nor should we even try. The world has changed. The gods change along with humans, and humans adjust theology and ethics to suit the needs of the times. One might say the Goddess is evolving, physically as well as symbolically, as the "unmanifest" of Her imaginings continue to manifest as the ever-changing universe. Yet I would argue that the wisdom inherent in the "old religion," the original pantheistic world view of Goddess cultures, is pertinent to the ethical (survival) dilemmas of our times; such an ethos makes us responsible to the universe for all our choices, individual and collective; to the survival of all species, including our own.

Works Cited

Ashe, Geoffrey. 1992. *Dawn Behind the Dawn: A Search for the Earthly Paradise*. New York: Henry Holt and Company.

Baring, Anne and Jules Cashford. 1992. *The Myth of the Goddess: Evolution of an Image*. London: Penguin Books.

Eisler, Riane. 1987. *The Chalice and the Blade: Our History, Our Future*. San Francisco: HarperSanFrancisco.

Eller, Cynthia. 1995. *Living in the Lap of the Goddess: The Feminist Spirituality Movement in America*. Boston: Beacon Press.

Luhrmann, T. M. 1989. *Persuasions of the Witch's Craft*. Cambridge, MA: Harvard University Press.

Starhawk. 1989. *The Spiral Dance: A Rebirth of the Ancient Religion of the Great Goddess*. San Francisco: Harper & Row Publishers.

Stone, Merlin. 1991. *Ancient Mirrors of Womanhood: A Treasury of Goddess and Heroine Lore from Around the World*. Boston: Beacon Press.

Chapter 2

The Circle of Life: Affirming Aboriginal Philosophies in Everyday Living

Laara Fitznor

The purpose of this paper is to highlight some of the complexities and struggles apparent in asserting Aboriginal philosophies, to highlight some of the philosophies inherent in Aboriginal[1] thought and, in spite of the struggles involved in asserting Aboriginal philosophies, to illustrate the visions that have been realized within Aboriginal contexts. To set the framework for this paper, I share some critical thoughts on writing about Aboriginal philosophies. Next, I discuss some of the struggles and complexities we as Aboriginal people experience in attempting to live the philosophies. Following this, I share some of the philosophies inherent in Aboriginal thought. Finally I share some visions and realizations wherein these philosophies can be celebrated. I caution the reader to appreciate the limitations of writing such an important piece of work: alas only some of the many facets of Aboriginal Philosophies[2] can be discussed in such a short space of time and place without compromising the rich and varied body of wisdom thriving in Aboriginal thought.

I write this paper by drawing on teachings[3] (knowledge and wisdom) from Elders[4] and educators (called traditional teachers) proficient in working from Aboriginal thought and oral traditions, and by drawing upon my own experiences. As I write this work, I acknowledge and appreciate the time and care one needs to take to acquire an in-depth knowledge and practice of Aboriginal knowledge and philosophies, whether or not one shares that identity and heritage. I make this statement in light of the times in which we live as Aboriginal peoples intricated in two worlds: a Western centric dominance and an Aboriginal heritage regaining, reclaiming its center.

On writing about Aboriginal Philosophies

I write this paper with the awareness and appreciation that many of our traditional teachers and elders are reluctant to write or record teachings.[5] These teachings are considered sacred and in need of protection from those who could take the knowledge and wisdom out of context and use it in an inappropriate manner where the cultural and spiritual life of Aboriginal peoples, the life of the earth and all life related to her, are threatened. Particularly, many people who work with the teachings are concerned that these teachings may be used against them again; examples of which have already transpired in colonialist Canada's history, such as making some of the traditional ceremonies criminal.

Also, traditional peoples have expressed concern that the value and significance of the oral nature of the traditions might be jeopardized in the process of documentation, where people will forget how to practice a tradition that is rich in its oratory.[6] An excellent memory and the concentration of heart and mind are required to be able to recite and relate the many intricacies involved in the oral traditions. The belief in the sacredness and protection of the oral teachings is so profound that many teachers of the teachings are reluctant to put words to paper.

As I suggest earlier, some of this reluctance to record any teachings is due to the wave of colonial oppression that sought to undermine any cultural, spiritual, or ceremonial event that occurred in Canada before the 1960's. A current public and political event that illustrates this reluctance to record took place during the proceedings of *The Royal Commission on Aboriginal Peoples*, where people were asked, in order to respect the integrity of the traditional ceremonies, not to record unless they received prior consent of the elders present.

However, as noted by some elders and writers, the time may be right to write from our perspective and on our own behalf. How fitting it is for our times that this reticence to write about our teachings is changing somewhat in some areas, particularly amongst Aboriginal writers and scholars who believe that it is time to start acknowledging Aboriginal philosophical perspectives, in a culturally and spiritually relevant manner. According to Couture, "It is true that the Elders who 'know' have been reticent, most discreet about sharing and teaching their 'knowledge.' However, those same Elders now point to an unfolding prophecy, which states that 'the time has come to share the secrets'" (Couture, "Explorations in Native Knowing," 54).

Many Aboriginal writers discuss the need to return to the teachings and the Elders. They state that to return to who we are as a People distinct and valid in our cultures and philosophies, we need to regain confidence in ourselves and in our teachings, not only for ourselves but for others seeking another way of looking at the world that is gentle and respective to the earth. Sharing these teachings in text form is one way to go. Couture notes that now that "most of the barriers to secrecy have fallen away, it is possible to access . . . some aspects of the characteristic content and mode of Native thinking, and to accede thereby to some of its power" ("Explorations in Native Knowing," 55). Likewise, Beverly Hungry Wolf discusses the need to write down some of the traditions of her grandmothers in order for learning and understanding between people to happen.

As I venture to write this work, I write with the hope that I may do so without compromising any of the traditions: I am writing to honor my people, all of life and oral traditions and in the hopes that this writing will reach a readership not normally versed in Aboriginal traditions. I hope also that those who read this will take these points seriously and with respect.

As I write this paper, I acknowledge and give thanks to the Creator for all of life and all the gifts we have received to sustain the healing, wisdom, and strength in mind, body and spirit. I acknowledge and give thanks to the Creator for this opportunity to create, to give, to share, and to live in a healthy way. I follow the lead of elders and traditional teachers who, when they start a teaching, begin by saying: "this was told to me, this is what was given to me, I was asked to pass this on, I acknowledge the many teachers I have had and I thank them for these teachings that I share with you." In this way, elders and traditional teachers are careful to not set themselves up as experts. Rather they acknowledge their ongoing learning about the teachings. Therefore, I share with you, the reader, the teachings that were 'given' to me, what I have been told about the teachings, what I have observed, and what I have read. However, I caution the reader that although I am Cree, versed in our traditions, in many ways I am a beginner in tuning into and drawing on Aboriginal Philosophies as a whole because I live in a "white world." Living within, beside, "in the face of," the dominant culture, and living in an urban setting, make opportunities for a fully Aboriginal thought and (social, personal, cultural, spiritual) life the daily struggle of affirming our differences against the framework of Western centric dominance.

Struggles and Complexities

Asserting Aboriginal Philosophies is a daily struggle because of the differences between the two worlds and because the "white world" has the status of legitimacy in North American society. As Aboriginal People, we struggle to gain any form of recognition for who we are as a people, let alone acknowledging and validating any ideas we might have about life. Imagine the struggles and complexities inherent in attempting to gain recognition and validation of our philosophies and perspectives. Many readings of historical pieces written from a critical and Aboriginal perspective describes these struggles clearly. Carol Locust notes:

> There is a long history of misunderstanding of Indian beliefs on the part of the dominant culture. Early, widely referenced scholars . . . seem to have assumed that American Indians were pagans (had no religion) or that they worshiped idols, animals, or devils. Such misunderstandings may have occurred because these scholars did not know the language or the customs of the people, and therefore interpreted Indian ceremonies from the perspectives of their own religious backgrounds. (Locust, "Wounding the Spirit," 316)

A rough road we travel, no doubt. Hence, the thoughts, themes, and words I use in this writing are shared because of my love and respect for, and belief in, the responsibility of our teachings.

It is important to dispel the notion that all Aboriginal Peoples, regardless of where we live, follow our original traditions or speak our languages to the fullest extent. The practices and reflections on these practices vary amongst our people. Due to the insidious nature of colonialism and the historical and contemporary stronghold of Christianity over Aboriginal Peoples, there are many people who have been influenced by Western centric faiths (particularly Christianity) so much so that this becomes their main practice, although there may be reliance on some of the traditions. Where the opportunity exists to integrate our philosophical, cultural and spiritual traditions, the practice of integration is more apparent. Another point to consider is that when Aboriginal people begin to return to the teachings, many experience conflict between the two world views and confusion about their identities becomes apparent during this process. In this sense a lot of healing needs to occur in the reclaiming process. Yet, in spite of these conflicts, Youngblood aptly states: "Still we passionately and intuitively seek the sacred realms, cultural restoration, and integrity: they are part of our humanness as Aboriginal People, a part of our consciousness and identity" (Youngblood, "Linguistic Rights in Canada," 13).

Consider the status of Aboriginal peoples: there are over one million Aboriginal People in Canada; over 2000 Aboriginal Communities in every province and territory. Aboriginal people live in cities; they live in primarily white rural settings; they live in mostly Aboriginal settings like First Nation's communities but ones primarily controlled by white governments and bureaucracy; they live in mixed White, Metis, and Status Indian communities. All of this makes full functioning of Aboriginal philosophies and practices difficult to achieve. We need to be aware of the complexity of the Western centric dominance and have an appreciation for the fact that there are many struggles involved in focusing energies and scarce resources to challenge stereotypes and problematic social conditions (suicides, incarcerations, chemical addictions, poor housing, poverty, high drop out rates, etc.), let alone in having the space to assert our perspectives in a culturally and spiritually relevant way supported by wisdom and knowledge of the oral traditions. Nevertheless, inroads are being made in all these areas.

The traditional world view of Aboriginal Peoples has been misunderstood and misrepresented, and many attempts have been made to interpret it through Western modes of thought, particularly through the Christian religions. It is important to note that I am not challenging Christian beliefs per se, but only the way Christian-focused organizations have sought to destroy the cultural, spiritual, and emotional sense of what it meant/means to be Aboriginal (some examples from Canadian history include residential schooling experiences, government controlled reserves, white controlled and administered educational and social programs).

Through this colonization process, the full essence of Aboriginal perspectives has tended to be distorted. Cajete, a Tewa American Indian and an academic, points out that though many of our people have succeeded within the "tradition of the American dream and all that it entails. . . . Indian People must question the effects modern education has had on their collective cultural, psychological, and ecological viability" (Cajete, *Look to the Mountain*, 22) and Indian People must consider what has been lost or gained by participating in a system that did not, does not, honor the essence of their philosophies. Clearly, Eurocentric thought paradigms continue to overpower our traditions in a way that puts the assertion of Aboriginal Perspective in continual struggle. Couture, a Metis-Cree Canadian and scholar, notes that we "from within our Native struggle . . . affirm ourselves now, *as we are*" (Couture, "Explorations in Native Knowing," 55). The disruption to our way of life that came from the process of colonization and oppression must be, and is being, stopped—though this occurs slowly. It would be remiss on my part not to note that alliances are forming to challenge continual colonization and oppression of Aboriginal perspectives, and that these come from all walks of life, including from many whites who see the Aboriginal way of life as valid and who see the need to respect and sustain Mother Earth and all her relations. We are working within a time frame where, as Aboriginal Peoples, we are asserting our rights in all facets of living: we are demanding lands to be restored to us; we are advocating that our philosophies and perspective be included in society, schools, educational processes; and we are demanding that our cultures be protected, and our rights to self-determination be recognized.

The timing may be right for us as the environment is in a state of crisis and, in recognition that Western modes of developing and industrializing are becoming less sustainable, many people are looking to us for answers. There have been, and there are, many prophecies inherent in the teachings/philosophies that speak to the history of what has happened and what is to come. These prophecies reflect a common theme: "The Earth is our Mother. We must take care of her" (Peterson, *Native American Prophecies*, xvi). By not taking care of her, as she sustains all of her people and life, we stand to lose more than we think. So we look to, listen to and trust in our prophecies. However, more trust and confidence in who we are as a people must first come from us as we appeal to the wider world to share the same confidence and trust in us as a people. Then we can advance the essence and truths of our knowledge for the sake of a future of safety and protection of the environment inclusive of all life.

Toward Understanding Aboriginal Philosophies

What do I mean by philosophies? In this paper, I mean the ethics of the people, the way people live, and their consciousness of living a way of life. For example, in Aboriginal thought, our philosophies carry a shared belief, a responsibility, a perception that is inclusive of nature, both material and spiritual, in the most intimate and interactive way. The relationship of the physical and spiritual world to our minds, bodies, and spiritual selves is reflected in this idea. Following this thought, Locust notes that:

> belief systems are the framework upon which cultures and societies function. It is the bond that holds civilizations together, and it is the small voice inside each of us that urges us to be true to what we have been taught. As Native people, we cannot separate our spiritual teachings from our learning, nor can we separate our beliefs about who, and what we are from our values and our behaviors. (Locust, "Wounding the Spirit," 328)

Youngblood also talks about world views as holistic constructs in which the past, present, and future and the environment are meshed. "World views strikes us as a big thought, as well it should. At first glance, it includes the entire known world. Yet, World views are limited" (Youngblood, "Linguistic Rights in Canada," 3). Further, Youngblood argues for the value of understanding how our world views are influenced by our indigenous languages. Aboriginal Peoples do have a world view, a way of coming into knowledge and looking at the world.

Pam Colorado, an Oneida woman, traditional teacher, and academic, notes that the words of various traditional teachers are reflections of "Native Science" (sic), which she refers to as "a way of coming to knowledge" of the truths and philosophies that act as guiding principles for living a life that has a "sacral basis" and that stems from teachings that "are grounded in the natural world." Still others attempt to identify Aboriginal thought as grounded in elder teachings, oral traditions and/or ceremonies such as the sweat lodge ceremonies, teaching circles, talking circles, healing circles, and the simple act of smudging for purification, giving thanks and acknowledging the Creator's gifts.

I began this section by noting that shared beliefs are shared across Aboriginal Peoples. However, it is important to acknowledge that diversity exists in languages, cultures, and spiritual practices, of different groups. How each of the teachings is taken up is defined by the personal experiences, the life, the land, regional ways, and culture of the group. The meaning of a teaching is also normally bound up with the cultural way of life of the teacher. For example:

> Traditionally, in the transmission of the oral tradition, the storyteller shapes the narrative with elements of their own cultural knowledge. Usually the audience shared the same cultural backgrounds, so the storyteller did not need to analyze each element or component of the story. (O'Meara and West, *From our Eyes*, 123)

Today, however, one will find that elders and traditional teachers tend to take more time to explain and analyze each element of a story, particularly if the people coming into the teaching circle are new to the situation. The respect for the place and time of each individual is usually acknowledged due to the conflict related to the dominant society's influence over Aboriginal thought. Deloria notes that diversity indeed is the norm though there are shared philosophies. He states "that there is no single Native science, each . . . Nation follows ways specific to a locale." The aspects of traditional philosophies that are universal/common include the "search of balance, harmony or peace with all living relations" (Deloria, *Red Earth White Lies*, 5).

Having noted the complex nature of our being as Aboriginal Peoples existing alongside a white world (our diversities and our similarities), let me share with you some of the philosophies as I understand them. I remind my reader that limited time and space do not permit me to go into depth in any of these areas, and that I deliberately choose only those that I feel I can share (based upon my experiences and some literature in the field) and those I feel will not compromise the sacredness of the oral traditions.

An important point to note is that, in contemporary society, working with the teachings automatically includes discussions about our personal and collective historic experiences with colonialism, racism and oppression, displacement of cultures, loss of Aboriginal languages, and experiences with residential schools among other things. I have witnessed many teachings taking place within a framework that addresses our being implicated in the dominant society. Sometimes, speakers of the teachings acknowledge and challenge the dominant society's influences that deprive many of our people of the details of their original teachings. Understanding the dominant society thus becomes part of traditional teaching; for example, when we note what happens when the Earth is not respected, or what happens when people are not respected. So on to some of the philosophies.

One of Canada's Ojibway Elders, Art Solomon, an Anishnawbe Spiritual Teacher who recently passed on when he was well over 80 years of age to the world of our ancestors, left his mark and his teachings with many of his followers. I am honored to have been present in many of his teaching circles. One of the main tenets of his teachings is noted in a book of poems and essays edited by Michael Posluns and titled *Songs for the People: Teachings on the Natural Way*. Contained in his poems with the teachings are lamentations about the devastation Aboriginal people have experienced at the will of white dominance in Canadian history. He acknowledges the healing process we must all experience. Our elder Art Solomon has said: "Everything that we do comes from the source of the Natural Law" (Solomon, *Poems and Essays*, 98); we are told that the creator has given much through Mother Earth's bounties so that people can live in wellness through healing, and wisdom. Solomon taught that all the Mother's bounties are like gifts and medicines, medicines that sustain us in times of plenty and heal us in times of need. He reflects on the notion of our responsibility, not only to the present but to the future generations, the responsibility of caring for Mother Earth and her people:

> We were the "Keepers of the Land" for the ones to come after us. We were to keep it in trust for them and we were to keep it clean and not disturb its harmony or its cycles because it belonged exclusively to the One who created and maintained it. And we, his [sic] children were only visitors here in this part of the creation. We were guests and we were to conduct ourselves in a sacred way. (Solomon, *Poems and Essays*, 98)

Colorado and Cajete also assert this principle of relationship with the natural world. Both note that we cannot separate ourselves from the land, the trees, the plants, the minerals, the rocks or anything that makes up part of Mother Earth. When we perceive the earth to be an interactive and living soul that has a consciousness, we tend to relate to her in a different manner than by attempting to control her resources only for our own use.

Another major principle reflective of Aboriginal thought is that of individual responsibility, relationships with others and the environment, and the significance of living the teachings in the fullest way possible. This idea is taken up in different ways in ceremonies, talks, healing circles, etc. For example, Bruce Elijah, an Oneida from Ontario, and an elder and spiritual teacher with whom I have had the honor of working in a teaching team, says that the notion of taking personal responsibility for one's "inner environment" is an essential requirement of working within the greater whole. This concept connects with being responsible in a reciprocal way. He says that each individual must first learn to live life from within a healthy inner environment in mind, body, spirit before s/he can understand fully the responsibility to the whole. This means working to understand one's personal imperfections and working toward a greater whole where conscious learning, relearning and healing, both for the person and for the community, takes place in mind, body and spirit. For Bruce Elijah, individual responsibility means living the teachings, even as we grow in understanding them, and even as they are reflected back to us. This is one of the keys to living fully in an Aboriginal world: me–you, we give and we take what we can with what we know and we work with it in an interconnected way for the healing of our outer environment.

The emphasis for Bruce Elijah is on learning, relearning and living the teachings, where much thought is given to developing critical thinking, to conscious working through of the principles, to building a conscience and ethics about a way of living and a way of looking at the world that is reflective of responsible knowledge, and of caring, giving, healing, and honoring the Creator in each and every one of our relations. Especially in today's world with the crises of our earth and its people, we need to work through this responsibility even more. Cajete's words reflect this consciousness:

> traditional American Indian education historically occurred in a holistic social context that developed the importance of each individual as a contributing member of the social group. Tribal education sustained a wholesome life process. It was an educational process that unfolded through mutual, reciprocal relationships between one's social group and the natural world. This relationship involved all dimensions of one's being, while providing both personal development and technical skills through participation in community life. It was essentially a communally integrated expression of environmental education. Understanding the depth of relationships and the significance of participating in all aspects of life are the keys to traditional American Indian education.
>
> Education is, at its essence, learning about life through participation and relationship in community, including not only people, but plants, animals, and the whole of nature. (Cajete, *Look to the Mountain*, 26)

Couture echoes these thoughts on relationships: "In traditional perception, nothing exists in isolation, everything is relative to every other being or thing" (Couture, "Explorations in Native Knowing," 59). Couture also notes that it takes a lifetime to grasp the full meaning of this reality. This is one theme that I have heard many times in many different talks, ceremonies, and gatherings. This theme reminds me of the times I have heard elders admonish those people who appear not to take what they are learning in a serious and respectful way, and those people who give the impression that they can learn everything faster through readings and sitting in only a few circles.

Interconnectedness, connections between everyone and everything: this is another philosophical theme that resounds throughout the teachings. The theme is expressed in various acts of living and honoring of life in ceremonies. For Aboriginal peoples, ceremonies are designed to honor the philosophies. In these ways, values are expressed to demonstrate and to deepen the knowledge of the complex web; all living things are imbued with sacred meanings. These thoughts/ideas are inherent in many sayings and teachings of Aboriginal Peoples. All of life is like this: mountains, prairies, plains, rivers, lakes, oceans, skies, animals, plants, insects, rocks, people are inseparably interconnected.

One of the key aspects of traditional knowledge is that there is spirit in everything, a notion that the Western mind may find difficult to perceive as reality. The earth (Mother Earth) and her inhabitants, the plants, animals, minerals, rocks, insects, etc., are all viewed in an interactive way—they are viewed as alive, as having a spirit, as conscious, and as capable of responding to people. They are our "relatives." In ceremonies and teaching circles each of these relatives is discussed in relation to its connection and contribution to the healing, wisdom, power and teaching of people. Each is given some instruction for us to live by. "The sacred powers of the four directions are still following their original instructions" (Solomon, *Poems and Essays*, 92) and we are all connected to these instructions in many ways.

One of the most interesting ways I have witnessed the meaning of working with the concept of interconnectedness and connections is the act of gathering the cooled ashes from one Sacred Fire, placing them in safe keeping, and later taking and offering them to a future Sacred Fire.

Building and working by a Sacred Fire (fire built for the purpose of healing and honoring sacred and oral traditions) promotes an atmosphere of trust and openness to learn and to work at our inner healing, and at all times we must remember our connections to others in a holistic sense, to come to what Colorado calls "truth in an Indian way," "truth that involves spirit, body, mind, and relationships" (Colorado, "American Indian Science," 16). Bruce Elijah shares this story. A Sacred Fire was built on Alcatraz Island during a reclaiming of the Island by Aboriginal peoples of the area and Aboriginal peoples from across Canada and United States who came to support this act of resistance. When the people were on the Island, they started a Sacred Fire which they nurtured to burn all the time they were there, twenty-four hours a day. Once the events stopped on Alcatraz Island, the people gathered the cooled ashes and took them to their respective communities and offered them in the next Sacred Fire each had visited. From then on each person continued to gather cooled ashes from each Sacred Fire only to take them to the next fire. For Bruce Elijah, this act was repeated many times over since the days of Alcatraz Island in the early 1970's. The teaching contained in this story demonstrates that we are all connected, and that the power is in the ashes—in the act of knowing and doing for the purpose of healing, support, and empowering. Now, I also repeat this act and when I do I am reminded of the hard work people put into their learning, healing and struggles for self-determination, and I am reminded of the continual connections of events from Alcatraz Island to now. In this way I have become interconnected with people that I do not even know but with whom I share a cultural and spiritual affinity. Finally, there is the constant acknowledgment of the connection to the natural law and to the notion that all that is, is related.

Working in settings where the teachings are shared, one can find many symbolic "objects" that are considered as our "relatives" and used in various ceremonies or sharing circles. The teachings reflected in these relatives include the acknowledgment of the four directions, the earth, and all living things on earth including what are inanimate from a western perspective. The interconnectedness amongst these is honored—it is as if one pays tribute to these relatives and their respective teachings throughout one's daily living. For example, when a ceremony is conducted, one can see that medicines (in Western terms, herbs and plants) will be drawn upon to help with the healing, to give wisdom and strength to the people. An eagle feather (the idea that the eagle's spirit holds significance is reflected here), and the teachings that the eagle feather brings, may be used in a sharing circle as a teaching tool and as a talking stick.

The idea that people need growth in many phases and spheres of their life is acknowledged in ceremonies. Everyone needs healing. Healing is not seen as simply about curing physical pain. It is seen in the more holistic sense of our need for continual guidance in our emotional, physical, mental and spiritual growth. All of earth's life forces, such as the four directions, have meaning and instructions from the Creator to guide us through life. In sharing knowledge many values are taught, among them: respect, love, sharing, honesty, and courage. These philosophies reflect a symbiotic relationship.

One of the key aspects of traditional knowledge, as I noted earlier, is that there is spirit in everything alive. So when plants, animals, minerals, and rocks are discussed, they are considered to have a consciousness and to be capable of responding. In this sense, the life of each element is as important as that of a human being. Traditionally when plants are taken from the earth, there is a discussion (prayers) with the Creator where the acknowledgment of one life giving to another is noted and appreciated. As noted earlier, each symbolic element is discussed in relation to its contribution to the healing, wisdom, power and teaching of all. Thus the elder may refer to a shell made from a turtle as the gift she, turtle, gave us. Couture outlines the importance these symbols have in teachings:

> journey symbols, heroic personalities, symbol of quartered circles, mandala symbolism of the self, various transformative symbolisms, the Great Mother, creation myths, initiation ceremonies, sacred pipe, sun dance, ghost dance, vision quest . . .The primal "experience" embraces the inner and outer worlds . . . In sum, traditional Indian knowledge is an experience in matter and spirit as inseparable realities. (Couture, "Explorations in Native Knowing," 58–59)

Visions and Realizations

Educators immersed in Aboriginal perspectives have long recognized the need for Aboriginal perspectives to have a place in the education system in particular. In this way Aboriginal people will regain the confidence almost lost in the colonial shuffle of cultural and racial oppression. As Hampton states:

> this new circle must encompass the importance Indian people place on the continuance of their ancestral traditions, respect individual uniqueness in spiritual expression, facilitate an understanding within the context of history and culture, develop a strong sense of place and service to community, and forge a commitment to educational and social transformation that recognizes and further empowers the inherent strength of Indian people and their cultures. (Hampton in Cajete, *Look to the Mountain*, 27)

The challenge then is how to put into practice this new circle of living when the perspectives have all but been lost. Devastating social conditions still dominate the lives of many Aboriginal Peoples to the point that many of our youth attempt suicide and many are unfortunately successful at committing suicide. How does our ethics deal with this problem? If the belief we hold is that life is precious, and that we hold value and significance as Aboriginal people, and that we have good and valuable philosophies that are acknowledged and validated within the dominant culture, and that we are connected to each other, that we are all related and all have a responsibility to each other's healing and growth, then we need to be able to communicate these beliefs to our youth. Incorporating Aboriginal philosophies by way of the healing circles, working with elders, working in ceremonies, ensuring that the symbolic "relatives" are used openly in education and public institutions without shame and without being ridiculed as being 'paganistic'—these are necessary first steps. Our youth need to be re-integrated into the Aboriginal circle of life with pride and honor while living without the pain of racism, rejection and the alienation they experience from conflicts in the dominant culture. Working with Aboriginal professionals, educated in Western centric colleges and universities as teachers, social workers, professors, physicians, and lawyers, is one way to help with the process of healing our people. Many of these professionals now attempt to include an Aboriginal perspective in their work, but they are met with resistance more often than not. We must find a way to work with elders and traditional teachers who can help in this process of re-integration for those of our people who are afraid to take this step.

Sharing circles used in public institutions are one example of putting into practice one aspect of Aboriginal traditions. Currently, there is beginning to be extensive use of the sharing circles for a number of areas such as teaching, working through conflicts and personal issues, working on healing and personal growth issues, working with the Aboriginal oral traditions, problem-solving techniques, and gathering critical information to help resolve issues. Therefore, at this stage, I will provide an explanation of how the Aboriginal tradition of sharing circles can be used.

Michael Hart discusses the value of utilizing the practice of sharing circles for teaching and supporting. He notes that: "the sharing circle has been used for many years by First Nations peoples as a format for communication, decision making, and support" (Hart, "Sharing Circles," 59). Although the notion of sharing circles is not evident in Western research paradigms, it is nevertheless important to Aboriginal traditions in Manitoba, when, for instance, people gather for the purpose of learning, sharing, and discussing issues and concerns.

Sharing circles embrace such concepts as learning from one another, and learning from what is said, gaining information and knowledge to incorporate into one's life, honoring and respecting what is heard, honoring the confidentiality of who said what, sharing the joy and pain of others, recognizing that what each person says is placed on an equal footing (no one person's voice is more important than an other's), and the willingness to share information about one's experiences in light of personal growth and development. Sharing circles promote personal well-being and the well-being of Aboriginal Peoples. They reflect the traditional concept of interconnectedness. Hart points out that:

> The sharing circles can establish dignity and unity by following the basic teachings of being holistic, in balance, connected, and in harmony. . . . Sharing circles are holistic in that everyone can participate. (Hart, "Sharing Circles," 59)

Therefore, although sharing circle practices may differ from region to region, or from cultural group to cultural group, many of the practices include the following:

(1)   Everyone is seated in a circle facing each other. A notion of equality is central here where everyone is considered to share an equal place in the circle of learning.

(2)   The topic at hand is placed, symbolically, at the center of the circle.

(3)   A designated leader (could be elder, group leader, teacher, etc.) opens the circle with a welcome, and explains the process for the circle. Often, but not always, a "prayer" and "smudging" occurs where the smoke from burning sweet grass is used in the circle. When sweet grass is used, usually each person sitting in the circle will "bath" themselves in the smoke to clear the eyes, ears, hearts, and mind, thereby getting rid of negative energy and opening themselves to positive energy (Hart, 68). The act of praying and smudging is primarily to give thanks to the Creator for life, and to ask participants to keep an open mind and heart for the task at hand.

(4)   Once the beginning stages of the circle are finished, often, but not always, a traditional sacred symbolic artifact[7] such as a stone, or an eagle feather is passed from left to right so that each person who speaks also holds the artifact. When individuals hold the object they can speak as little or as long as they feel it necessary to do so: the "person is free to speak as long as the object is held" (Hart, 68). In addition to this process, if the group leader feels it is necessary, once each person has had the time to say his or her piece, the object is then placed in the center of the circle and if people want to add to what was already said they can. In some practices, if this is done "Anyone wishing to speak must pick up the object" (68) but this practice is not always the same. Often when this process is used people can add to what they said because of hearing someone else make a point. It encourages more ideas and experiences to be recalled.

(5)   Once the circle is complete, the group leader takes the last position of speaking and, depending on the purpose of the circle, s/he thanks each

person for what was shared, and may add some words of encouragement, and some thoughts on future actions resulting from the circle work. Sometimes, individuals are reminded, at this stage, of the concepts and philosophies governing sharing circles. They are then asked to honor these important "teachings" as they leave the group.

(6)   Finally, before anyone leaves the circle, people demonstrate their appreciation, trust, understanding, and honor of each other's viewpoints by staying in the circle for a handshake or hug. The leader starts off and gives a hug or a handshake to each person to his/her left, the next person follows, and the next follows that individual. This action continues until each person has given, and received, a handshake or hug. The connections between people are demonstrated in this way.

Including an Aboriginal perspective within western paradigms by means of sharing circles can be done in a classroom in certain cases. It is important to note here another Aboriginal tradition, that of using tobacco in significant transactions such as asking for an Elder's help, or asking people to get involved in an Elder's healing, and promoting the well-being of others. The tobacco is considered a traditional "medicine" and it is used for healing, praying, teaching, and working. According to Aboriginal traditional teachings, "tobacco is 'the first plant' given by the Creator, thus its use in ceremony" (Hart, 68) and its use in interactions for healing and teaching. It is symbolic of the opener of good thoughts, good interactions; it communicates honor and understanding of Aboriginal perspectives in the interaction.

Opening a circle with a "ceremony" helps the students gain information about the philosophies behind cultural and oral traditional Aboriginal thinking. Another purpose of the ceremony is to allow students to experience the practices related to the teachings.

Finally, I will share with you what I have observed as some of the medicines that have been used in sharing circles. I would like to acknowledge Jules and Margaret Lavallee for these teachings acquired through their learning over the years. They were clear about stating this acknowledgment of learning from other Elders as I asked for their permission to write these up as I heard and observed them.

(1)   Tobacco can be used regularly when using the Sacred Pipe in a sharing circle. One of the sacred medicines, tobacco is used for prayers and requests, and thanksgiving. Tobacco is used regularly to open any event that has a healing, learning, or teaching significance attached to it. It calls

for clearing minds and hearts and for one to be open to the knowledge being shared for the purpose of learning, to live life to its fullest potential, spiritually, mentally, physically, and emotionally. All of the teachings in some way contribute to this purpose. It is also important to acknowledge the significance of the Sacred Pipe as it is generally used with Tobacco. The pipe represents peace, reconciliation, humility, and purification. The Sacred Pipe "is assembled in prayer, offered to the four directions, the sky and earth . . . [to] promote clear thinking . . . The smoke symbolically transports us, our prayers and requests to the Creator" (*All My Relations*, 19).

(2)   Sage can be used for smudging. This occurs when the Elder instructs that each person clear him/herself with the smudging. Sage is normally placed in a traditional bowl of a natural element, such as a sea shell, and set to smoulder. One of the students who acts as an Elder's helper then takes it around the circle. Each participant cups the smoke in his/her hands and bathes him/herself with it by pushing the smoke toward their bodies with their hands. It is explained that if people do not feel comfortable with the smudging they do not have to smudge themselves.

Sage is used most often in the healing circle, sharing circle and traditional circle. It is usually recognized as being a Woman's Medicine; therefore it can be used to honor the women in the group.

Water is usually part of every opening circle. This is also recognized in traditional circles as representing Woman's gift.

(3)   Sweet grass is braided in three strands to honor mind, body, and spirit. In traditional teachings sweet grass provides positive energy, good thought, honor, and purification. This is one of the sacred medicines. Sweet grass represents Mother Earth's hair. In ceremony, a smouldering braid of sweet grass is taken around the circle gathered. Each participant cups the smoke in his or her hands and bathes with it. "The smoke from the sweet grass promotes positive energy and good thoughts, so that the group's purpose remains clear, and the result benefits the people" (*All My Relations*, 19).

(4)   Cedar can be used in the Smudge Ceremony during the opening of the circle. Cedar, in a symbolic way, deals with resolving conflicts.

(5) Weekay is another Medicine that can by used by the elder. Weekay is considered our Spirit Medicine. Placing weekay in one's mouth is an acknowledgment that the Spirit guides one's words and actions.

Conclusions

Meegwetch (Ojibway), *Ekosi* (Cree). I give my acknowledgment of "thanks and appreciation," first in the Ojibway language then in the Cree language to those relatives and Elders who have been my teachers, and to those brothers and sisters who have been my traditional teachers for all the words I have shared in this paper. I give acknowledgment to the numerous authors who have taken the courage to write about these perspectives—they have helped me to develop this paper as I have attempted to share how I interpret Aboriginal Philosophies. I am reminded daily that in spite of the struggles and complexities that are prevalent in our lives as Aboriginal people, we can look toward thriving in the new circle of life by celebrating our philosophies in every which way we can, and by asserting ourselves through more harmonious interaction and connection with all of our relations. *Ekosi.*

Notes

1. The term "Aboriginal" used in this paper (also the term "Native" when cited) includes all Aboriginal groups (Metis, Status Indians, Non-Status Indians, and Inuit) in Canada, and the United States. Writers from the United States tend to use the term Indian in the generic sense. Many Aboriginal Peoples from the older generation still tend to use the term "Indian" in a generic sense. However it is falling out of usage, particularly once people realize that it is a legal definition that does not include all Aboriginal Peoples. Readers are reminded that complex diversity of languages, cultures, and traditions thrive amongst the Aboriginal groups. For example, in Manitoba alone, there are five cultural/linguistic groups. Although, there are common threads to Aboriginal thought, the living context dictates differences in practices.

2. Aboriginal Philosophies embrace a multi-faceted, multi-layered, multi-culture of traditions, beliefs, and ideas. This paper only skims the surface of what is there and what can be discussed without undermining the integrity of the knowledge and the reasons for living the knowledge (the practices). Only a few of the themes that are more commonly shared and openly practiced are discussed here.

3. The term "teachings" used in this paper refers to the knowledge, wisdom, sacred secrets, and truths shared by the Aboriginal way of coming into knowledge about the relationships in all of life and nature. "Teachings" is a term that is commonly used amongst Aboriginal Peoples.

4. According to Couture, the term Elder is used for those individuals who believe in teaching, following and sharing the Aboriginal way of life and in reclaiming and asserting our sense of Aboriginal identities. Usually Elders are older people, though some are younger people who would be perceived as traditional teachers, versed in the knowledge and wisdom and striving to live life to its fullest. Elders are, as Couture states, "The exemplars of such a way of living, relating and perceiving . . . [they] . . . are superb embodiments of highly developed human potential" ("Explorations in Native Knowing," 209). In contemporary society, elders are people living in two worlds: for some this type of existence continues to be a struggle to maintain balance and to ensure that their voices (teachings) are heard in spite of the Western centric framework that implicates us all.

5. I have been a participant in many ceremonies, circle teachings, and in many discussions with elders where the idea of taking notes or recording what was heard and said is highly suspect. However, many Elders now acknowledge that the time is right to begin sharing the sacred teachings, particularly if this is done in a "good way," i.e., to help the environment (Mother Earth) and all her relations (people, plants, animals, insects, minerals, etc.).

6. I have discussed the nature of the oral traditions with Jules Lavallee and Margaret Lavallee, a husband and wife team, both Ojiway and traditional teachers, and elders. Jules emphasizes that his work as an elder and traditional teacher necessitates that he remember the detailed and intricate knowledge and wisdom contained in each symbol, song, story, and dance. For example, it might take anywhere from a few minutes to a few hours to orate the main message and wisdom conveyed in just one symbol.

7. Calling these items artifacts is really a misnomer from the perspective of traditional Aboriginal Peoples, because each of these items is believed to contain a living spirit, e.g., our ancestors who have passed on and have come to guide us in our daily lives.

Works Cited

All My Relations: Sharing Native Values Through the Arts. 1988. Compiled by Catherine Verrall in consultation with Lenore Keeshig-Tobias. Toronto: Canadian Association in Support of Native Peoples.

Bobb, Judie, Michael Bobb, Phil Lane, and Carolyn Peter. Special Edition, 1988. *The Sacred Tree.* Lethbridge, AB: Four Worlds Development Project, The University of Lethbridge.

Burger, Julian. 1990. *The Gaia Altas of First Peoples: A Future for the Indigenous World.* New York: Anchor Books, Doubleday.

Cajete, Gregory. 1994. *Look to the Mountain: An Ecology of Indigenous Education.* Durando, CO: Kivaki Press.

Colorado, Pamela. 1988. "American Indian Science." Paper Presented to the 46th Congress of the Americanists, Amsterdam, Holland. July 4–8.

Couture, Joseph. 1991. "Explorations in Native Knowing." In *The Cultural Maze: Complex Questions on Native Destiny in Western Canada,* edited by John W. Friesen. Calgary, AB: Detselig Enterprises Ltd. 53–73.

———. 1991. "The Role of Native Elders: Emergent Issues." In *The Cultural Maze: Complex Questions on Native Destiny in Western Canada,* edited by John W. Friesen. Calgary, AB: Detselig Enterprises Ltd. 201–217.

Deloria, Vine, Jr. 1996. *Red Earth White Lies: Native Americans and the Myth of Scientific Fact.* New York: Scribner.

Elijah, Bruce. 1997. Oneida Elder, Personal communication. March, July and September.

Ermine,William. 1995. "Aboriginal Epistomology." In *First Nations Education in Canada: The Circle Unfolds,* edited by Marie Battiste and Jean Barman. Vancouver: University of Brititsh Columbia Press.

Hart, Michael Anthony. 1996. "Sharing Circles: Utilizing Traditional Practise Methods for Teaching, Helping, and Supporting." In *From our Eyes: Learning from Indigenous Peoples,* edited by Sylvia O'Meara and Douglas A. West. Toronto: Garamond Press.

Hungry Wolf, Beverly. 1980. *The Ways of My Grandmothers.* New York: Quill.

Knudtson, Peter, and David Suzuki. 1993. *Wisdom of the Elders.* Toronto: Stoddart Publishing Co. Limited.

Lavallee, Margaret and Jules Lavallee. 1997. Ojibway Elders. Personal communication, July, September.

Locust, Carol. 1988. "Wounding the Spirit: Discrimination and Traditional American Indian Belief Systems." In *Harvard Educational Review* vol. 58 no. 3: 315–330.

O'Meara, Sylvia, and Douglas A. West, eds. 1996. *From our Eyes: Learning from Indigenous Peoples.* Toronto: Garamond Press.

Peterson, Scott. 1990. *Native American Prophecies: Examining the History, Wisdom and Startling Predictions of Visionary Native Americans.* New York: Paragon House.

Report of Royal Commission on Aboriginal Peoples. 1996. Volumes 1 to 4. Canada Communication Group Publishing.

Solomon, Arthur. 1992. *Poems and Essays of Arthur Solomon, A Nishnawbe Spiritual Teacher - Songs for the People: Teachings on the Natural Way.* Edited by Michael Posluns. Toronto: New Canada Press Limited.

Youngblood, James [Sakej]. 1993. "Linguistic Rights in Canada: Collusion or Collisions? Governing the Implicate Order." Paper presented at University of Ottawa, Faculty of Law, Friday, December 31.

Chapter 3

Buddhists Within the Moral Space of Non-Duality

Eva K. Neumaier

The Buddhist traditions are grounded in the experience of one human being, Gautama, who received the title Buddha, the Awakened One, after he had an irreversible mystical experience, i.e., he awoke to an insight which, he believed, liberated him from the ongoing cycle of dying and being reborn. Gautama lived in India, approximately 2500 years ago. As a truth seeker he certainly had absorbed some of the major ideas of his time while he did not claim divine descent or to be god reincarnated.

Textual evidence points to the effect that the community of his followers embraced, at least in large parts, common assumptions about the salvific nature of a life of moral restraint. To limit the amount and kind of food one would consume, the hours spent sleeping, the intensity and frequency of social contacts, these and similar restrictions seemed to the early Buddhists to provide the best conditions for a fruitful pursuit of realizing the awakening their leader had pointed out to them. A life of restraint (in Sanskrit *shila*, "discipline") was seen as a necessary basis for a life devoted to meditation and the acquisition of wisdom. Together, morality, meditation, and wisdom formed the major building blocks of an eightfold soteriological path that promised the achievement of enlightenment. The numerous precepts which constituted the Buddhist code of ethics were based on the opinion that they would facilitate the realization of enlightenment, which—at least in theory—was the goal of all Buddhists. Only the authority of the Buddha was invoked to back up the authenticity of the precepts.

I would like to lay the foundation of this contribution by summarizing the normative side of Buddhist ethics, that is, to survey what the texts say about how an ideal Buddhist should act. From there I move on to examine the lives of some exemplary Buddhists and raise the question of how their actual behavior was in accord with the ethical norm of the belief they had embraced. As we shall see, the findings are mixed, ranging from an ancient emperor who was a truly moral person to other dignitaries whose acts and words were far apart. The final section will discuss two major figures of contemporary engaged Buddhism: Dr. Ambedkar, the advocate of the Untouchables, and Thich Nhat Hanh, the Vietnamese Buddhist monk and political activist.

Normative Ethics

Like other founders of major religious traditions, the Buddha has not left behind any written records. The collections of his discourses (in Sanskrit *sutras*), as memorized by his disciples, were put into writing before the beginning of the Common Era, but systematic discussions of the Buddhist doctrine did not appear for another four to five hundred years.

One such systematic discussion is attributed to Buddhaghosa (fifth century CE), a monk, originally from India, who became the main tutor of the form of Buddhism which came to dominate the South East Asian countries (usually referred to as Theravada[1]); its title is *The Path to Purity.*[2] This work, which is praised as a comprehensive commentary on the entire Pali Canon,[3] or, according to others, as an encyclopedia summarizing its main ideas, is organized in three sections: ethics, meditation, and wisdom. In his treatment of ethics, Buddhaghosa sees the five precepts (abstention from killing any living thing, from stealing, from sexual misconduct, from lying, from slanderous or hurtful talk) as basis for the development of higher ethics expressed in the hundreds of rules guiding the lives of monks and nuns. Religiously well motivated lay people may follow three or five more precepts in addition to the mandatory five ones for a given time or for the rest of their lives. These additional rules include abstention from social entertainments as well as the renunciation of comfort and luxury and the rejection of mind-affecting substances (such as, alcohol or nicotine). Without exception, Buddhaghosa emphasizes mental restraint and discipline as the major aspects which make moral action possible. It is the lack of egotistic desire as well as the cultivated equanimity with regard to the social and material world which makes one an ethical person. The mechanical avoidance of prohibited acts has little merit in this system of thought. According to Buddhaghosa, the withdrawal of the senses from the world must be a major concern for monks and nuns as only then the mind may find stillness and will become pure—crucial conditions for the path to enlightenment. To contemplate the fragile and mortal nature of the human body, so the text assures its readers, will safeguard the monastic person against all temptation of lust and passion. The issue of how acts of high morals may affect the other person (may this be a suitor or a former spouse or other relative) is not asked. This issue will only occasionally be raised within some Mahayana texts.[4]

While the pre-Mahayana Schools of Buddhism see ethics as ancillary to a contemplative life and the pursuit of wisdom, the Mahayana Schools see compassion as *the* proper activity. The unenlightened individual has to make an effort to act out of compassion and needs to engage in specific meditations to condition one's mind accordingly. But the enlightened individual, one who has become a Buddha, will find compassion to be his or her natural way of acting. In some Mahayana texts it is said that all acts are grounded in the buddha-nature of reality and are therefore acts of compassion, regardless how these acts may be seen by an unenlightened person. But this compassion has to be paired with wisdom which has transcended egotistic concerns. Consequently this compassion does not judge between right and wrong, or innocent and guilty, but knows of the interdependence of all that exists.

Exemplary Lives

In the past, the exemplary was usually invested in members of the elite. This observation is also true with regard to the Buddhist traditions. Among the exemplary lay people Emperor Ashoka (reigned from 273 to 232 BCE) stands high above others. His patronage of Buddhism transformed "a local sect into one of the world-religions" (Smith, *Oxford History of India*, 117). Ashoka left behind extensive testimonies to his world view, his motivations and his ethics by inscribing his thoughts on rock pillars or rock surfaces. His policy of peace, inspired by a sincere commitment to Buddha's teachings, became a yardstick for assessing the ethics of any later Buddhist ruler. Ashoka announced, in number XIII of the Rock Edicts, his motivations for pursuing politics of peace:

> Kalinga was conquered by His Sacred and Gracious Majesty when he had been consecrated eight years [261 BCE]. 150,000 were thence carried away captive, 100,000 were there slain, and many times that number died. Directly after the annexation of the Kalingas began His Sacred Majesty's zealous protection of the Law of Piety, his love of that Law, and his inculcation of the Law (*dharma*). Thus arose His Sacred Majesty's remorse for having conquered the Kalingas, because the conquest of a country previously unconquered involves the slaughter, death, and carrying away captive of the people. That is a matter of profound sorrow and regret to His Sacred Majesty. (Smith, *Oxford History of India*, 119)

Buddhist ethics, with their emphasis on peace and non-violence, altered the behavior and style of government of one of the most powerful monarchs India had known in its long history. Instead of further embarking on campaigns of conquest, he confessed his wrongs publicly, hence pursuing a policy of peace-making and non-violence. For Ashoka, true conquest was then the conquest of people's hearts by the Buddhist doctrine. Therefore, he devoted much of his reign to the promotion of Buddhism and made Buddhist ethics the basis of his government and of legislations.

Despite the fact that Ashoka was unanimously praised by Buddhist traditions as an exemplary virtuous ruler, other Buddhist rulers followed different standards. The Dalai Lamas, secular rulers over Tibet since 1642 and embodiments of Avalokiteshvara, the bodhisattva of immeasurable compassion, are such an example. The religious rank of the Dalai Lamas rests upon the claim that the bodhisattva of ultimate compassion, Avalokiteshvara, embodies himself every time in them.[5] Thus, so is professed, the rule of the Dalai Lamas is guided by compassion.

As members of the Gelugpa Order,[6] the Dalai Lamas saw themselves as entrusted with the task of creating a social and cultural situation most suitable for the practice of Buddhism in general and for the advancement of the Gelugpa order in particular. The fifth Dalai Lama was most instrumental in shaping these conditions. To achieve this goal, he enlisted the help of Gushri Khan, his Mongolian patron, to overthrow (and later execute) the patron of his opponent, the leader of the Karmapa Order. Thus, by depriving his religious foe of secular protection, the fifth Dalai Lama was able to establish his power and become the first of the Dalai Lamas to assume the title "King of Tibet." Religious sophistry would find it of course quite possible to reason why this act of violence was necessary and "good" as it served a higher purpose, i.e., to establish the rule of the Dalai Lamas which, so the claim goes, eventually provided the most beneficial circumstances for the practice of the Buddhist religion (understood here as a practice based on the Gelukpa tradition).[7]

One may argue that this had happened in the seventeenth century, a time when perceptions of ethics and morality were quite different from today's, but similar discrepancies can be detected in the behavior of the officials of the Tibetan government of our time too. A case in point is the execution of Lungshar, a Tibetan aristocrat serving under the thirteenth Dalai Lama. He had been sent to England "with power to discuss matters for the benefit of Tibet."[8] Soon he became acquainted with key events of European history, such as the French Revolution and the concomitant execution of many of Europe's monarchs. Upon his return to Tibet, Lungshar attempted to reform the feudalistic structure of Tibet's government by changing the lifelong appointments of cabinet ministers to a four-year term (Goldstein, *History of Modern Tibet*, 190f). On the day he was about to present his reform plan to the cabinet, a junior official denounced him of conspiracy and of plans to annex the country. As a consequence of this unverified allegation, Lungshar was imprisoned. After a short trial, he was condemned to death by the investigating committee. But "it feared that someone as willful as Lungshar might become a vengeful ghost . . . they recommended . . . mutilation—in this case, the removal of both eyeballs" (207). The cabinet (which included secular officers beside clerical ones) agreed to this punishment "but Reting (the regent, a high ranking monk who lead the government during the interregnum between the thirteenth and fourteenth Dalai Lamas) tried to avoid responsibility by telling the Kashag (the Tibetan cabinet) that it would not be proper for a lama (high ranking Buddhist teacher) and Gelong (Buddhist monk) to sign a mutilation order" (208). Instead the regent told the cabinet ministers that they should see to it, meaning that they should carry out the verdict without the regent's signature on it—so it was done. The operation was botched as for some time the punishment had not been inflicted on anyone. The result was that one eyeball was pried out while the other had to be cut out with the help of a knife (208f). The present Dalai Lama expresses his appreciation for Reting Rinpoche, the regent who had approved Lungshar's mutilation, by saying that "despite his mistakes, I still retain a deep personal respect for Reting Rinpoche as my first tutor and *guru*" (Dalai Lama XIV, *Freedom in Exile*, 31). As a sign of his respect for his tutor, the Dalai Lama restored Reting Rinpoche's name to the name list of his spiritual ancestry.

In reflecting on negotiations with leaders of the People's Republic of China, the Dalai Lama reveals his own moral philosophy: "I believe that the most important thing for humankind is its own creativity. I further believe that, in order to be able to exercise their creativity, people need to be free" (Dalai Lama XIV, 242). Obviously, Lungshar's reform plans were not considered to be creative and, thus, he did not deserve freedom—but mutilation. Nevertheless, "[a] future free Tibet will seek to help all those in need . . . and to promote peace" (Dalai Lama XIV, 271).

The apparent duplicity in these cases may, to some degree, be caused by the fact that the actors were holders of political power, that proclamations of their Buddhist belief remained disconnected from their acts. Critical as one may be of such lack of integration, it is not uncommon among people of power and authority. But what about humble Buddhists whom the tradition later elevated to an exemplary status? Such a person was without any doubt Milarepa. Born into a peasant family near Mt. Everest in the eleventh century, he may be seen as a magician, a great poet, or a saint. As an adolescent he exhibited a disconcerting temper, but throughout his life he preserved an air of innocence which sometimes bordered on the bizarre. His main fascination however was with being and acting as enlightened being. Thus, his behavior was often not in accord with common norms and values as he acted from a vantage point of enlightenment rather than convention. Thus, Milarepa reveals quite a different side of Buddhist ethics (Bacot, *Milarepa*, 17–19).

Only one incident, told in his life-story, shall suffice to make the point (Lobsang, *Life of Milarepa*, 138f). For some time Milarepa had lived in the mountainous wilderness at the foot of Mt. Everest. In solitude he lived mainly on wild plants and seeds and slowly his simple clothes disintegrated so that he was nude. When his sister visited him, she felt ashamed of his nudity. She reprimanded him that such behavior was inappropriate for a holy man, in particular as his genitals were exposed. On her next visit she brought a piece of fabric so that Milarepa could sew some clothes for himself. Instead of doing what was expected of him, i.e., sewing proper clothes which would correspond to the feelings of decency and shame of his culture, Milarepa cut the fabric into small pieces and made small covers for all body parts which "stuck out"—nose, fingers, and others. When confronted with the accusation that his behavior violated Buddhist perceptions of modesty, Milarepa answered that there was nothing to be ashamed of because he had received his entire body, including the offensive parts, from his parents.

Humorous as the incident is, it makes the shallowness of conventional morality visible. While Milarepa was surely not in support of immodesty and exhibitionism, he showed in this incident that common feelings of modesty were rooted in the visual, and often unadmitted, pleasure of gazing. The body parts *per se* were not immodest but the gaze and its desire were immodest. Consequently, if his sister found his nudity immodest, the true immodesty was her desiring gaze.

Milarepa exhibited here a behavior similar to that reported of some Zen masters who challenged conventional perceptions at the risk of being offensive in order to evoke liberating insight among their disciples. I shall come back to this issue of ethics transcending morality in my concluding paragraph.

Buddhist Ethics in Response to Contemporary Culture

The cases of Buddhist ethics discussed so far derive from texts written many centuries ago or from pre-industrial cultural contexts, and, one may ask, "What about ethics in contemporary Buddhism?" As Queen and King in the introduction to their study of contemporary reformist movements in Asia said, "Buddhism in contemporary Asia means energetic engagement with social and political issues and crises" rather than introspective withdrawal (Queen and King, *Engaged Buddhism*, ix). Hence I shall discuss the social activism of Dr. Ambedkar who saw Buddhism as a social and humanistic philosophy to liberate the deprived and oppressed, and contrast it with the teachings of the Vietnamese Buddhist master Thich Nhat Hanh.

Queen presents Dr. Ambedkar as typifying the "modern man" in so far as Bhimrao Ramji Ambedkar (1891–1956) was born into the certainty of ancient Hinduism but opted as an adult for Buddhism to free himself and others from circumstances he deemed oppressive (Queen, "Dr. Ambedkar," 45–71). Many reviewers of Ambedkar's main works on Buddhism criticized him for altering Buddhism so that it became unrecognizable. Ambedkar's Buddhism was unrecognizable to Buddhists brought up in century and millennia old Buddhist traditions and to scholars who, in all regularity, are more concerned with the history of Buddhist thought and texts rather than with a lived religiosity. But Ambedkar's Buddhism aroused hopes and faith in many millions of Indians who, born as Untouchables, vegetated at the fringe of a society torn by social and political unrest and upheaval.

The pivotal teaching of Buddhism, i.e., the four noble truths, say that life is suffering, that it is caused by a thirst for being, that if this thirst can be extinguished nirvana will be achieved, and that there is an eightfold path to realize this goal. Traditionally this teaching resulted in an emphasis on meditation, a monastic or reclusive lifestyle, and in seeing the cause of suffering within the person who suffers. As I have said elsewhere, traditional Buddhism psychologized the suffering of individuals as well as of communities (Neumaier-Dargyay, "Feminine Perspective," 151). As long as the cause of suffering is seen as lying in the person's past activities and desires, no incentive for social action is provided, or, that at least is how Ambedkar saw it. This individualistic trend became most visible among the various pre-Mahayana Schools which advocated that each individual has to work out his or her enlightenment on their own. The Mahayana Schools limited this trend in so far as they saw the realization of enlightenment as an act which can only happen in a universal context. While the goal of Buddhism was universalized in Mahayana, the same did not happen with suffering which remained within the scope of the individual's responsibility despite being the basis for the path to nirvana and enlightenment.

Ambedkar based his rethinking of Buddhist thought on three premises: rationality, social benefit, and certainty. He deemed authentic only those canonical statements which he saw in accord with these criteria. In his reading of Buddhist teaching, he rejected the traditional explication of the four noble truths, of karma, and nirvana, to name only a few examples (Queen, "Dr. Ambedkar," 59).

One might assume that Ambedkar reasoned that the message of the Buddha must make sense to the Untouchables of India and, in a larger context, to all oppressed people. The intentional simplicity and poverty of the traditional Buddhist monastic person must appear as a frivolity to those who lived in systemic and structural poverty. The *karma* theory which, to put it bluntly, "blames the victim" for the endured pain offers the Untouchables little in terms of emancipatory tools. To the contrary, the *karma* theory could paralyze emancipatory desires and moves among the oppressed as these acts would only lead to increased suffering if one accepts the traditional reasoning.

Ambedkar did not use the traditional interpretation of Buddhist texts as a guideline for his own understanding of Buddha's message, instead he looked at Buddha's resourcefulness as a teacher "who sought to encourage the individual disciple's ability to think for himself" (Queen, 60). Queen argues convincingly that Ambedkar presented a fresh interpretation of the Buddhist teaching which, in its essence, was less radical than some of the statements of the Perfection of Wisdom sutras. Consequently, Ambedkar dwelled extensively on the inclusion of women and outcastes among the Buddhist monastic order. He detailed that not only women of Buddha's own noble family found acceptance there but also Untouchable ones, as well as prostitutes and serial killers. Thus, Ambedkar suggested, one can see how the Buddha broke class and social barriers to establish all humanity in a society of security and equality, in other words, in a state beyond suffering.

Ambedkar's Buddhism transfigures ancient Buddhist concerns to fit into a modern context, and uses contemporary language to do so. There is "the reality of human suffering, the availability of relief through self-cultivation and compassionate action, and the potential for a liberated society based on equality and opportunity" (Queen, 62). Thus, the first noble truth is understood as the widespread poverty and injustice of our time; the second one as the institutional and corporate greed, hatred and oppression, as well as the delusions so readily disseminated; the third truth (traditionally the assertion of nirvana) is seen in the light of the ideals of the European Enlightenment of "liberty, equality and fraternity"; while the fourth truth showing the path how to achieve this goal is contained in Ambedkar's call to "educate, agitate, organize!"

While traditional Buddhist ethics were designed to assist the individual to purify his or her mind as a condition for realizing enlightenment, Ambedkar's Buddhism saw in ethics, as defined by him, the primary means to establish a society which was constituted in equality and justice and, thus, free from suffering.

The moral responses articulated by Buddhists of Vietnam to the political and social challenges imposed on them by the colonial powers of France and the United States as well as by their respective ideologies resulted in a form of engaged Buddhism which is significantly different from Ambedkar's. Thich Nhat Hanh became "arguably the most important theoretician of this Vietnamese movement" (King, "Thich Nhat Hanh," 321). As one of the foremost minds of the Unified Buddhist Church his thoughts and actions inspired the church but, at the same time, not all the actions of all its members reflected Thich Nhat Hanh's views. Thich Nhat Hanh is a contemporary Vietnamese Zen master who, fully in line with the tradition of past Zen masters, uses poetry as a means to evoke reflection but also as a means to provoke activism.

When American intervention in Vietnam produced socio-political circumstances which made the practice of Buddhism increasingly difficult, Nhat Hanh and other committed Buddhists, monastics as well as lay people, strove to reverse this trend. Thus, their activism was initially re-active to government measures. However, as the war progressed with ever greater brutality and as the suffering of the ordinary Vietnamese peasant became more glaring, Nhat Hanh defined two goals for an engaged Buddhism: first, to eliminate or at least minimize suffering; second, to do so in a spirit of non-duality.

Both concepts need further exploration. The first concept, to eliminate or minimize suffering, is an enactment of the four noble truths: the first of which talks about the universality of suffering while the other three deal with the elimination of suffering. Unlike Ambedkar, who rejected the traditional explanation of the four noble truths, Nhat Hanh accepted them but applied them to the concrete socio-political situation of Vietnam. In practical terms it meant that monks and nuns in their bright yellow robes often formed a live barricade to separate the aggressors from each other or to protect peasants from their attackers. It meant to provide shelter and home for the many war orphans, to heal the wounds of the body and mind, to rebuild destroyed villages, and to provide education (King, 337).

The second goal was to place one's activism solidly within non-dualism. To understand this moral non-dualism, a closer look at Nhat Hanh's philosophy is required. In a poem, Nhat Hanh identifies himself not only with insects and reptiles but also with the raped girl and her rapist. At first sight, the poem may leave the impression that there is no good and evil, that killer and killed, prey and predator are on the same level of moral indifference. As a Buddhist, Nhat Hanh looked at the world not from a vantage point which sets the human species essentially apart from all other life forms but from a perspective of an all-integrating interdependence. Rape victim and rapist, prey and predator are players in the same game; both condition and define each other. Both are, in a way, enmeshed in the same net of desire and passion. If one were born under the conditions of the rapist, one would end up being a rapist. Thus, he, too, deserves compassion as he is not the autonomous doer he may seem.

As a consequence, Nhat Hanh avoided taking sides in the war. It was neither the North Vietnamese nor the South Vietnamese government he and his fellow Buddhists supported. Neither the Viet Cong nor the American soldier ought to be killed but the killing had to stop. "Please call me by my true names; I am the joy and the sorrow," Nhat Hanh says in his poem. "Through this identification with both good and bad, through meditative discovery of the impulses behind one's own 'goodness' and 'badness' one can finally put aside these categories and 'wake up,' opening one's heart to compassion" (King, 341).

In the non-dual activism of Thich Nhat Hanh, Buddhist ethics finds its purest articulation. While in the high moral standards of Ashoka a certain amount of self-righteousness is present where right and wrong are in juxtaposition, a natural compassion which embraces victim and perpetrator as being players in the same game is visible in the non-judging ethics of Nhat Hanh and his fellow Vietnamese Buddhists. The normative texts do not provide us with provocative images such as the one created by Nhat Hanh:

> I am the 12-year-old girl, refugee on a small boat,
> who throws herself into the ocean after being raped by a sea pirate,
> and I am the pirate, my heart not yet capable of seeing and loving.
> (King, "Thich Nhat Hanh," 339)

While the examination of the lives of some of the Dalai Lamas leaves us with an impression of duplicity, the life story of Milarepa throws a refreshing and at the same time penetrating light on conventional morals. By challenging conventional mores he, like some Zen masters, opens the possibility to transcend conventions and to find one's way to invoke one's own ethics, which, for the enlightened being are nothing but acting out of buddha-nature, i.e., compassion. The normative texts, however, seem to erect barriers and impose judgement where the lived ethics of some Buddhists breath the air of genuine compassion that embraces all living beings in their own suffering. This compassion, although rooted in mindfulness and meditation, is far from aloof introspection; it is the way of the Buddhas.

Notes

1. The naming of the various strands of the Buddhist traditions has recently undergone some changes. While in the past it was common to see Theravada as part of the Hinayana, the "lesser method," more recent publications introduced the term Nikaya Buddhism instead of Hinayana in order to avoid the derogatory label given by their doctrinal foes while at the same time acknowledging the multitude of sects and schools of which Theravada forms only one.

2. A discussion of the author and his work is found in K. R. Norman, *Pali Literature*, 120–30.

3. The Pali Canon contains works ascribed by the Theravada tradition to the historical Buddha as well as systematic explications of them. Some scholars see in the Pali Canon the oldest layer of Buddhist texts. For further information see K. R. Norman, *Pali Literature*.

4. The term Mahayana comprises a fairly wide diversity of Buddhist traditions which can be traced back to certain ideological and philosophical trends increasingly dominating the discourse among the Buddhist communities by the beginning of the Common Era. Ideologically they all endorse a more ahistoristic view of the Buddha, emphasize an understanding of mystical transmutation in immanence, and see the *bodhisattva* (a person directed by the desire to teach the entire universe how to realize enlightenment, i.e., a Buddha-to-be) as the most excellent religious hero. For further information see Paul Williams, *Mahayana Buddhism*.

5. Avalokiteshavara is a so-called "celestial" *bodhisattva* which means he is an allegoric being residing in a paradise-like imaginative place from where he radiates compassion throughout the universe. One day when all sentient beings are about to realize nirvana, Avalokiteshvara will then become a Buddha. Apparently early on in the course of Tibetan history, the myth of Avalokiteshvara became fused with a pre-Buddhist myth narrating the heavenly descent and the sacred nature of the Tibetan ruler. In the *Mani bka' 'bum* the classic narrative of this fused myth is found. The Dalai Lamas appropriated the myth when they became rulers over Tibet. For an account of the political aspect of the Dalai Lamas, see Tsepon W. D. Shakabpa, *Tibet: A Political History*. The Avalokiteshvara myth in relation to the rulers of Tibet is the subject of Eva K. Dargyay, "Srong-btsan Sgam-po of Tibet: Bodhisattva and King" in *Monks and Magicians: Religious Biographies in Asia*, 99–117.

6. "The ones on the virtuous path" understood themselves as a reform movement to curb laxities and abuses among the Tibetan monastic orders. About two hundred years after the Gelugpas' inception, the fifth Dalai Lama, already recognized as their foremost leader, became ruler of Tibet. See Melvyn C. Goldstein, *A History of Modern Tibet 1913–1951: the Demise of the Lamaist State*, 1.

7. The main events are detailed by Tsepon W. D. Shakabpa, *Tibet: A Political History*, 107–112.

8. Quoted from the translation of Lungshar's credentials in Melvyn C. Goldstein, *A History of Modern Tibet*, 159.

Works Cited

Bacot, Jacques. 1974. *Milarepa: ses méfaits, ses épreuves, son illimination*. Paris: Éditions Robert Laffont.

Dalai Lama XIVth (Bstan-'dzin-rgya-mtsho). 1990. *Freedom in Exile: the Autobiography of the Dalai Lama*. New York: Harper Collins.

Dargyay, Eva K. 1988. "Srong-btsan Sgam-po of Tibet: Bodhisattva and King." In *Monks and Magicians: Religious Biographies in Asia*, edited by Phyllis Granoff and K. Shinohara. Oakville, ON: Mosaic Press.

Goldstein, Melvyn C. 1991. *A History of Modern Tibet 1913–1951: the Demise of the Lamaist State*. Berkeley: University of California Press.

King, Sallie B. 1996. "Thich Nhat Hanh and the Unified Buddhist Church of Vietnam: Nondualism in Action." In *Engaged Buddhism: Buddhist Liberation Movements in Asia*, edited by Christopher S. Queen and Sallie B. King. Albany, NY: State University of New York Press.

Lobsang, Lhalungpa, trans. 1977. *The Life of Milarepa*. New York: E. P. Dutton.

Neumaier-Dargyay, Eva K. 1995. "Buddhist Thought from a Feminist Perspective." In *Gender, Genre and Religion: Feminist Reflections*, edited by Morny Joy and Eva K. Neumaier-Dargyay. Waterloo, ON: Wilfred Laurier University Press.

Norman, K. R. 1983. *Pali Literature (History of Indian Literature,* vol. 7, no. 2*)*. Edited by Jan Gonda. Wiesbaden: Otto Harrassowitz.

Queen, Christopher S. "Dr. Ambedkar and the Hermeneutics of Buddhist Liberation." In *Engaged Buddhism: Buddhist Liberation Movements in Asia*, edited by Christopher S. Queen and Sallie B. King. Albany, NY: State University of New York Press.

Queen, Christopher S. and Sallie B. King, eds. 1996. *Engaged Buddhism: Buddhist Liberation Movements in Asia*. Albany, NY: State University of New York Press.

Shakabpa, Tsepon W. D. 1967. *Tibet: A Political History*. New Haven: Yale University Press.

Smith, Vincent A. 1981. *The Oxford History of India* (4th edition). Oxford: Oxford University Press (First published in 1919).

Williams, Paul. 1989. *Mahayana Buddhism: The Doctrinal Foundations*. London and New York: Routledge.

Chapter 4

The Life-Ethics of the Bhagavadgītā as Interpreted by Rāmānuja

Klaus K. Klostermaier

"Life ethics" is a modern concept based on fairly recent Western cultural pre-suppositions rooted in Greek, Christian, Humanistic, and increasingly, in legalistic notions of "value." Life-ethics issues in Western countries are today closely tied to economics: a cost-benefit calculus is usually the *ultima ratio* for decisions in this area. In other cultures the philosophical and the legal bases are sufficiently different to make it difficult, if not impossible, to transfer present Western notions of life ethics. We have to remind ourselves that also in the West thinking on these issues in the past differed radically from country to country, and from one historic period to the other. The notion of a universal life-ethic is closely linked to the notion of universal human rights as declared by the United Nations in 1946. The declaration assumes the existence of an egalitarian "human nature" inherent in all human beings, and rights associated with that human nature that are universal and non-negotiable. Recent attempts to articulate a global ethic go one step further in that direction. Comments from countries like China, which reject Western complaints about human rights violations in their jurisdictions, go some way to show that not all are agreed on what human rights mean and how far individual rights can be maintained over against larger social claims and necessities.

Historic instances preceding the UNO declaration of universal human rights are not lacking that attempted to establish specific cultural norms as a universal standard for human behavior. Thus the ancient Greeks assumed that their own ethic (*aretai/virtues*) formed the divide between human and non-human: those bipeds that did not share Athenian behavior were mere animals, without "human rights." Furthermore, it was anyhow assumed that only humans had rights, and often only specific humans: males, wealthy individuals, persons born into a certain class or caste, etc. Similarly the people accepting the Bible as the very Word of God took the observation of the Ten Commandments, upon which the Biblical Covenant was founded, as the dividing line between the "children of God" and the others. The "others" were usually exposed to considerable disadvantages and certainly were not seen as possessing universal "human rights." The treatment meted out by the Israelites to the Canaanites, and then by the Christians to Jews (relying on a further "new" covenant) was not only an expression of popular sentiment but was supposed to be justified by divine command. Hindus and Buddhists, as well as Jains, believed that their own code of behavior was *sanātana dharma*, eternal, universal law. While Buddhists and Jains believed in persuading people to accept this *dharma*, Hindu society enforced it quite rigorously. Full humanity was only conceded to the *Āryas* who lived according to the *varnāśramadharma*—the others were called *mlecchas* (people with an unacceptable language) or *nispriyas* (untouchables), no-bodies.

It is obviously very difficult to match the notions of "ethic" and "dharma": they are governed by different presuppositions, different societal structures and different interests. It is on that background that we are dealing with the "life-ethics" of the Bhagavadgītā. It requires us to read the text from an "ethics" perspective that is alien to the Indian tradition of which it is part. Many modern Hindus use the Gītā as their "Guide" and attempt to extrapolate from it guidelines for their behavior in today's world. This paper will first deal with life-ethics issues raised in the Bhagavadgītā and then examine how Rāmānuja has commented on these issues.

The Life-Ethics Teachings of the Bhagavadgītā

The Gītā calls itself a "Yogaśāstra," a text designed to reach ultimate union with the Highest, and each chapter individually deals with a particular kind of *yoga*.[1] It is traditionally considered a "Dharmaśāstra," a text supporting and elucidating *dharma*. As Duncan M. Derret has pointed out, *dharma* is not the result of theoretical or logical conceptualizations but of experience lived through several generations and interpreted in the spirit of these experiences. It is very malleable and beyond the grasp of outsiders who do not share this experience. It is group-centered and group-oriented. It is based on notions of authority, duty, consensus. It is in many ways the very opposite of "ethics" as understood in the modern West with its emphasis on individual rights and equality.[2]

According to the widely accepted *Manusmrti*, humans are born with five debts which define their place in the world: all have innate duties towards god(s), towards ancestors, towards elders/parents/teachers, towards fellow human beings, and towards non-human creatures. Life is meant to be spent redeeming these debts. This is done through worship, remembrance of dead ancestors, support of parents and teachers, hospitality, and care for animals and spirits. In addition, according to the caste one is born into, each human has specific (caste) duties to fulfill: the brahmin's duty is to teach, the kṣatriya's duty is to fight and to rule, the vaiśya's duty is to procure the necessities of life, and the śūdra's duty is to supply labor. While part of the fulfilment of duties no doubt goes towards the maintenance of society and state (*lokasaṅgraha*), the fulfilment of one's *svadharma* also guarantees transcendental blessings and fulfilment of a "religious" agenda.

Much has changed since the Bhagavadgītā was promulgated but its principles are still widely accepted as reflecting the Hindu ethos. Not only does it contain the *yama-niyama* rules (the Indian equivalent of the Ten Commandments) that are taken as universal norms for ethical behavior, it also contains the meta-ethical principles that allow one to solve more complex ethical dilemmas.

It clearly represents a "divine command ethic," insisting that the norm of (good) behavior is *vidhi*, i.e., scriptural injunction.[3] It also suggests that humans do not "make history" but are only actors in a play whose script has been written by God who also is stage-director, seeing to it that the play is proceeding according to the script, no matter what. This predeterminism is intrinsically linked with the theory of karma and the acceptance of *punarjanma* ("rebirth"). While the preservation of physical life seems to have become the highest medical ethical imperative (and the most lucrative industry as well) in contemporary Western culture in peacetime (in wartime the destruction of the maximum number of "enemy" lives seems to the highest "ethical" imperative!), the traditional Indian attitude, reflected also in the Gītā, is quite different. Given the overall high mortality rate, the suddenness with which death could strike down large numbers of people in catastrophes and epidemics, life was seen and accepted as precarious. The conviction that a particular life-span was only an episode in a long history of multiple incarnations of an indestructible *ātman* certainly gave a different perspective. There is no metaphysical reason to do everything to prolong a particular life since it is not seen as unique and is not believed to be the end of the existence of a particular person. The Gītā also is based on the notion of a Personal God as ultimate and saving Reality—personalizing what otherwise would be an objective Law.

When addressing "life-ethics" issues, the Gītā moves on two levels: Arjuna presents the traditional Vedic *dharma* which is apparently unable to address the situation. Kṛṣṇa reveals a higher kind of wisdom in whose light the insoluble dilemmas of the "old ethic" become irrelevant, even non-existent. Overall the Gītā replaces an ethical approach to life-problems by a metaphysic: what used to be seen as personal problems involving agonizing decisions fraught with uncertainty are declared to be mere phenomena of nature following their own impersonal laws. The personal dimension is shifted to a transcendent level: the only decision required for finding ultimate salvation is the surrender of one's will to God, the relinquishing of desire and the firm resolve to fulfill God's command.

The whole Bhagavadgītā deals with one "life-ethic" issue: the question of "just war," "holy war," killing and being killed. It presupposes that a war for the sake of defending and upholding *dharma* is just. It also presupposes that persons (men) belonging to the kṣatriya-caste (soldiers, administrators) have a religious duty to engage in such war and that for them dying in such a war is the surest way to "heaven," and that killing in such a war is no sin. The *ultima ratio*, and the basis of the entire "ethic" of the Bhagavadgītā is the preservation of *varṇāśramadharma*, which is understood as *sanātana dharma*, eternal law, ordained by the Creator, and indispensable for maintaining world-order. On that point it agrees with the "old" ethic represented by Arjuna. Its interpretation and reasoning, however, are different. The Gītā goes further than previous *dharmaśāstra* texts: it declares that also fratricidal wars (which were prohibited by traditional law and which were supposed to lead to the punishment in hells) could be made "just" if, over and above defending one's rights, they were fought in a "spirit of detachment," i.e., free from motives of greed and hatred.

Rāmānuja's Interpretation

The authors of the Gītā had presumably expected and hoped that their "reformation" would replace the old and no longer workable notions of *dharma*. While it certainly became popular it did not succeed in completely ousting the old thinking. When the Gupta restoration of Hinduism took place, it was first the Mīmāmsakas, and then the Vedāntins, who argued against and eventually defeated the predominant Buddhists. The Hindu renaissance included a revival of the ancient, pre-Gītā notions of *dharma*. The new champions of Hinduism had to take care to cover all bases and to address all adherents of Hindu *dharma*. Thus we find in some of the Gītā commentaries written by the champions of Vedānta opinions expressed on matters of *dharma* that the Gītā had left behind. In addition, they use the text of the Gītā as an occasion to promulgate their own thinking and to support the teachings of their *saṁpradāyas*.

Rāmānuja subscribes to the Gītā notion of *sanātana dharma*, the "naturalness" of traditional Hindu *varṇāśramadharma*, its God-given nature. As a Vaiṣṇava, he sees in *bhakti* the highest calling of a human person and reads the Gītā as a text that inculcates love to God as the first and foremost duty. As a Śrivaisnava he emphasizes *prapatti*, complete surrender to God as the proper attitude. From this it would follow that a human person would unconditionally execute every command understood to be divine.

Given the Gītā's clear (and necessary) emphasis on metaphysics over against ethics, it comes as a surprise to see Rāmānuja in his *Gītābhāsya* give a higher standing to *karma-yoga* (which he sees as the essence of *bhakti*, warning against (unqualified) jñāna-yoga as dangerous and an occasion for downfall. Jñāna-yoga, the condition of "contemplation," non-action, is, of course, no longer the subject-matter of ethics—there are no duties to be performed, no changes in the outward world to be effected.

As Aristotle advised not to teach ethics to young people, because they lacked the practical/political experience out of which ethics is distilled, so Rāmānuja (with most of the Hindu tradition) cautions not to teach the Bhagavadgītā "to someone who does not practice *tapas*, nor to someone who practices *tapas* but not *bhakti*, nor to someone who, though he practices *bhakti*, does not listen, nor to someone who discovers defects in God's proper form, his sovereignty and his virtues" (XVIII, 67 [174]).[4]

For Rāmānuja the purpose of the Gītā and the purpose of life is the cultivation of *bhakti*: "When the proper form of one's *ātman*, whose nature is to be a *śeṣa* of God and whose form is unlimited knowledge, has been revealed . . . one will not mourn over any being but God, nor desire any being but God, but be equal and indifferent towards all beings; not caring for anything, one will acquire *bhakti* towards God—supreme *bhakti* which is the experiencing of the most dearly beloved One" (XVIII, 54 [172]). When that condition is reached it entails a *bharanyāsa*, a surrender of all (ethical) responsibility to God himself:

One should leave all acts—together with agency and object—to God because one knows that one is ruled by God; and, while realizing that it is God who is to be attained, and in that spirit performing one's acts and devoting oneself to this buddhiyoga, one should always keep God in mind. Then, while being absorbed in God, and performing all acts, one will escape from all dangers of *saṁsāra* by the grace of God. When, however, one refrains from listening to God's word, because one thinks one knows everything that ought and ought not to be done, then one will be lost; for God alone knows what all living beings ought and ought not to do, and He is their law-giver. (XVIII, 57–58 [172f])

For Rāmānuja the purpose of Vedānta—*jñānaniṣṭhā* (preventing the senses from action) or *ātmāniṣṭhā* (steadfastness in the Self—is not identical with cessation of action but with the "accomplishment of disinterested activity meant to propitiate God" (III, 4 [67]). "One must be active" and "there is no existence without activity" (III, 5 [67]). He offers a practical reason for preferring *karmayoga* to *jñānayoga*: If one attempts to practice *jñānayoga* before the karma created by the gunas have been annulled by *karmayoga* "one would perish even while practicing *jñānayoga*. One must be active, because by nature one is conjoined to *prakṛti*" (III, 8 [67]). *Karmayoga* is more important than *jñānayoga* even for a person qualified to do *jñānayoga* because "in order to sustain his body a person has to be active in performing sacrifices and the like" and "*karmayoga* . . . does not cause a person to be negligent about it" (III, 8 [68]).

Being content with Self/God alone is the aim of all endeavor—thus someone who has reached that stage where "the ātman is everything—livelihood, nourishment, experience—need not perform the act prescribed for his varna and asrama." At that stage "contemplation no longer depends on either the means of release, *jñānayoga* and *karmayoga*. Such a person will turn away from all non-spiritual things of his own accord" (III, 18 [71]). There is no ethical necessity, because no action is prescribed to perform or to avoid.

The Gītā teaches that persons in leading positions, who may no longer need action in order to purify themselves from *karma*, have to act in order to give an example: "God is not bound to do anything, for there is no desire of his that is not fulfilled; yet He is active in order to save the world" (III, 21 [71]). Rāmānuja calls *svadharma* "a propitiation of God."

A man devoted to his proper task (according to varṇāśrama) attains the highest end . . . when by means of his proper acts he has worshiped God as the Inner Ruler . . . he will attain God, who is the cause of all activity of all beings and the pervader of the universe, by the grace of God. (XVIII, 45 [171])

As far as the actual events are concerned—what we used to call "history"—these are not the result of human decisions, ethical or otherwise, but are preordained. The human ethical freedom is restricted to accepting or not accepting as God's will what is going to happen.

All beings are forced by the Lord to follow their prakrti in accordance with their previous karma. The Lord Vasudeva who is wont to rule all, resides in the hearts of all beings—the heart from which arises all knowledge and on which all action and inaction depends—while actuating by means of his own *mā yā* all beings which are put in that mechanism which is called prakrti developed into body and senses. For this reason Arjuna should completely submit himself to God, the Lord of all. If not, he will still have to fight the battle, inevitably, for his ignorance stimulated by God's *mā yā*, will make him do so. Therefore he should fight the battle in the manner which God has explained; then God's grace will make him attain supreme Santi—the release from all bonds of all acts—and the eternal end. (XVIII, 60ff [173])

Most Westerners who have heard of Mahatma Gandhi associate Hinduism with the advocacy of *ahiṁsā*, non-violence. His "peaceful resistance" was admired even by US civil-rights leaders. *Ahiṁsā* is certainly not the message of Vedic Hinduism. It was introduced into Indian thought through the Upanisads and such heterodox movements like Jainism and Buddhism, which advocated abolition of the frequent animal sacrifices. Vaiṣṇavism integrated, amongst other elements, ahiṁsā into its practice: in Vaiṣṇava worship, only flowers, fruits and vegetables are offered to the deities. However, Vaiṣṇavism upheld the old orthodoxies with regard to the kṣatriya's duties and vedic sacrifice. Thus Rāmānuja insists:

> The annihilation of the body is a reason for joy, for when one has abandoned one's body in lawful warfare, then, so the *śā stras* assert, one will receive a beautified body in return; it is like throwing away one's old dress and putting on a new one. (II, 22 [56])
>
> Arjuna should look upon this warfare as his dharma, a dharma of the same order as that of agnisoma sacrifices. Such warfare is most salutary to a kṣatriya. The immolation of the sacrificial animal at agniṣṭoma sacrifices cannot be regarded as *hiṁsā*, for according to the *śruti* the victim, when having abandoned an inferior body—a he-goat, e.g.—will attain heaven with a beautified body . . . those who have been killed in battle will receive a more beautiful body in return; the immolation of a victim at rites such as *agniṣṭoma* sacrifices, is therefore not *hiṁsā*, but is actually a way of protecting the victim, and as such comparable to the treatment with a thorn by a physician. (II, 31 [57])

Rāmānuja concludes:

> Such warfare, which causes immeasurable bliss, is the share of none but a kṣatriya of good karma. If, in his ignorance Arjuna refrains, after having already begun, from waging the war which is his dharma, he will be deprived of the immeasurable bliss, which results from the observance of dharma and of the fame of victory; so he will gain nothing but evil. Moreover, everybody, expert or no expert, will cry shame upon him and that disgrace will be worse than death for a hero like him. It does not count that he refrains from battling because of his

love and his compassion for his relatives: such a thing does not happen and nobody will believe him; instead they will think that fear makes him do so. Then they will disparage his heroism: death is preferable to such disparagement.

Therefore, both alternatives, either that he kills his enemies or that his enemies kill him are to be preferred to his refusal to enter into battle: in the first case he will, when killed, participate in supreme bliss, and in the latter case he will enjoy his kingdom without rivals when they are killed, and moreover, enjoy supreme bliss because his *dharma*, if observed disinterestedly, will lead thereto . . . If one aspires to release one will wage war with the certain knowledge that the atman is different from the body, that it has nothing in common with corporeal nature and that it is eternal. . . . (II, 32 ff [58])

The whole argument rests on the premise that the human person is an asymmetrical combination of an eternal *ātman* (spirit-soul) and a mortal body and that, as far as bodily existence is concerned, the law of karma applies inexorably. Religion as a means to overcome the results of karma (of which rebirth is the most crucial!) is primarily a karma-yoga, i.e., a teaching of duties/actions that neutralize the effects of past karma and that prevents the accumulation of new karma in this life.

In a reply to the question as to why the Vedas prescribe acts that lead to new births and not to release, Rāmānuja counsels:

One should not accept all which is taught by the Vedas; just as a thirsty man does not take more water from a public reservoir than he is need of so a Vedic aspirant to release should not take more from the Vedas than his release requires. No more is required than this: when performing sacrificial acts which according to *śruti* leads to certain results, one should consider the act in itself reason enough to perform it, and not its result; for any result makes another tie, but resultless acts which are performed to propitiate God serve to release. Therefore one should not be oneself the reason of acts and results . . . one must not remain inactive but one must perform acts disinterestedly and with equanimity as to their failure or success. (II, 46 [61])

Rāmānuja therefore recommends to "apply the *buddhi* to one's actions," i.e., be conscious of the "proper form of the *ātman*"—such acts "take away all suffering in *saṁsāra* and further release" (the others "result in immense suffering in saṁsāra"). "When one applies this *buddhi* to one's actions one relinquishes the good and evil karman which has been collected in beginning less times, which has no end and which is the cause of one's bondage to *prakrti*" (II, 50 [62]). What he means really, is *bhakti/prapatti*:

He who does not focus his mind on God will not be able to form in his mind the *buddhi* that is concerned with the atman as distinct from prakrti, or to cultivate his knowledge of this distinct atman by meditating on it, or to subdue his propensity to the objects, or to obtain ever the eternal perfect beatitude. (II, 72 [65])

Every practice is a preparation for bhakti, which is an end in itself.

Knowledge of the *ātman* combined with *karmayoga* leads to *jñānayoga*; through *jñānayoga* one arrives at the true contemplation of the realized *ātman*. This contemplation, again, is propaedeutic to *bhaktiyoga*; through *bhakti* alone one is capable of attaining God. (II, 72 [65])

Rāmānuja lays stress on the fact that karma-yoga, in order to be "yoga" (i.e., a liberating/unifying activity) and not just "karma" (the performance of prescribed acts), must involve the knowledge that the *ātman* is distinct from the body (III, 18 [81]). "There are many ways of practicing karmayoga and all of them lead to true knowledge of the *ātman*. All of them result from periodical and occasional acts which are being performed day by day. When one knows and observes this, then one will be released" (III, 22 [83]). Pithily, Rāmānuja concludes the discussion on karmayoga by saying "karmayoga is worship of God" (III, 29 [91]).

The ethical model—the perfect karmayogi—is one who:

does not hate any being, even though it hates him. He is friendly to all beings, whether they hate him or help him. He is compassionate towards all beings which love him. He is not possessive and does not suffer under the delusion that his body is the *ātman*. So he is neither delighted nor vexed when fortune or misfortune befall him, for fortune or misfortune are only imagined. He is not transformed by rivalry and power even if they are inevitable. He is satisfied with whatever he may find for the sustenance of his body. He is constantly occupied by the thought that the *ātman* is different from *prakrti* . . . ." (XII, 13ff [135])

Our Western understanding of ethics—especially religious ethics—includes the assumption that acts that are "ethical" are the result of free choice: it implies that everyone has a choice to act or not to act ethically. According to Aristotle there can be no choice about actions which are intrinsically bad such as murder, theft and adultery. This philosophical assumption has been questioned in practice by psychologists and sociologists who often succeed in convincing judges and juries that certain acts were either done out of a compulsion, over which the agent had no control, or were attributable to the milieu in which an offender grew up. The Gītā holds—and Rāmānuja agrees—that people are predisposed to ethical or unethical actions by being born either into the family of God or into the family of the Demon. The former naturally would be generous, would fulfill their religious duties, be sincere, non-violent, tell truth "if the truth is not offensive" (XVI, 2 [155]), be free from anger, compassionate, patient and considerate. The persons of the other kind were "born to infringe God's commandments" (XVI, 3 [156]) and are conceited, irascible, ignorant of the Vedic *dharma* which leads to prosperity and release (XVI, 3 [156]).

Those who belong to the family of the demons lack the philosophico-religious insights and principles upon which ethic is built:

> They deny that the world is ensouled by brahman and that it is ruled by God . . . they do not realize that the ātman differs from the body and they lack all discernment. Consequently they do much harm to everybody: they are born to bring the world to ruin. . . . Trapped by a hundred hopes and acting upon nothing but desire and anger, they aspire criminally to many things in order to enjoy their desires. They are ignorant enough to think that they have obtained all they possess by their own efforts and not by virtue of an unseen cause. . . . They do not allow for an unseen factor . . . (XVI, 8f [157]). The demoniac nature has a threefold cause which destroys the *ātman*, viz. [namely] desire, anger and greed. (XVI, 8f [158])

If, as Rāmānuja does, the aim of life is seen in *mokṣa* and *sākṣātkāra*—life itself being considered an occasion to serve God—the resulting "life-ethic" is very different from an ethic that is intended to serve the hedonistic/materialistic aim of most contemporary Western people. Truly religious people have taken upon themselves many deprivations—for the sake of service of God and fellow men—that non-religious people would consider an infringement on their "right to happiness." While we may not be able to learn much detail for a "life-ethic" from Rāmānuja's interpretation of the Bhagavadgītā, it may make us reflect on meta-ethical issues and the meaning of life as a whole. While we may deplore the result of the ethical deliberation reached at in the Bhagavadgītā, namely the decision to begin the war that became known as the "Mahābhārata War," the most destructive war the world had seen till then, we must respect the effort to decide on matters of war and peace from a standpoint of ethic rather than power-politics.

For Rāmānuja it is not a question of finding a new societal consensus on acceptable personal behavior but it is a question of re-discovering the true meaning of the eternal law that has been promulgated before time and that guarantees both the continuation of society and the personal fulfilment of its members. From its very beginning and in its very structure this society and its ethic has been non-egalitarian. Within each of the *varnas* every aspect of life has been covered by detailed regulations. Nothing is left out and everything has to be done according to the existing rules. Interpretation of these rules was not left to each individual. On a local level there were Panchayats, councils of five, which regularly met and dealt with infringements of regulations. Nationwide, there used to be a Dharma Parisad, a religious authority, that was to interpret and adapt the *dharma* in changing circumstances. This no longer exists. Major figures, known as "Reformers," in the 19th and 20th centuries fulfilled the role in an unofficial manner. One of the last and most widely known such was Sarvepalli Radhakrishnan, a leading intellectual and statesman. He not only translated and commented on the entire *prasthāna trayī* but also considered his office as President of India as "conscience of the nation." He taught a liberal, enlightened, "demythologized" Hinduism and expressed himself, from a Hindu perspective, on many contemporary problems in India and world-wide. At present the more vociferous Hindus seem to be conservative, chauvinistic, reactionary. They advocate violence, if necessary, to win back dominion over India, they defend *satī* and restrictive legislation in many areas, they decry the corrupt West and feel morally superior. Nobody can say what they will do once they are in power.

"Life-ethic" in the Bhagavadgītā, as in all traditional "scriptural," institutional religions, means the submission of the individual's aims and actions under a universal "divine" schema or purpose. For the representatives of these religions, the existing institutions are the expression of the ultimate and everything must be done to preserve them. "Good" or "bad" are relative to this ultimate end: what contributes to the preservation of the (divinely instituted) order is "good," what is contrary to it is "bad." Individuals per se do not count; they count only as an embodiment of the "great idea" or as tools to reach the institutional aim. Thus the death of any number of individuals is justified as long as it promotes the divine purpose: the killing of the "enemies" of the Kingdom of God is a virtuous act; the death of defenders of the faith in their battle against the enemies is heroic and praiseworthy—it is not to be lamented but rejoiced in ("sanguis martyrum semen Christianorum"!)[5]. Any aspect of ethic—including life-ethic—is reduced to conforming with the established order: there are few problems to be solved and few new answers to be sought. Traditional ethic does not appeal to individual conscience but to collective duty. The primary purpose of traditional ethic is the maintenance and continuity of a particular order of society, not the preservation of an individual life.

Concluding Reflections

Reading about the religious war-rhetoric of World War I, in Deschner's *Ein Jahrhundert Heilsgeschichte*, it struck me how similar the argumentation is to that of the Bhagavadgītā. The Catholic bishops declare active participation in World War I a religious duty. It is "God's Will," and the war itself is seen as a divinely ordained cleansing of the world. They provide Christian arguments in order to overcome the inhibition to kill relations and fellow-Christians of other nations. It is amazing to learn that the decalogue injunction "thou shalt not kill" has now been overridden by a "war-imperative." It would be intriguing to write a Bhagavadgītā commentary with the words of bishops and preachers who supported World Wars I and II on both sides, and to compare their "after-war" rhetoric with the situation in the Mahābhārata after the war. It seems strange that theistic religions, which usually exhibit such rigorous positions when it comes to ethics of property or sexuality, could be so eager to fight wars "for God," to kill in the name of religion, and to believe that killing "enemies" is a virtuous deed to be rewarded by God in heaven. Is the clergy's instinct for power so overwhelming and so blinding that it makes them not even recognize the irony? Why should an Almighty God need politicians and military to pursue his aims?

Strange also the kind of illusionistic-idealistic expectations that war would bring about a moral rebirth and a "cleansing" of people, the expectation that somehow or other through those beastly doings God's realm would be established once and for ever. Anybody who has lived through a modern war will confirm that it is hell on earth, that it destroys not only lives and properties, but also minds and morals. Modern war is legalized mass-criminality perpetrated with the most powerful technological means available by hundreds of thousands of well-trained men and women. We rightly bemoan the loss of a single life in a senseless act of brutality, the loss of a home in a natural calamity, the trauma caused to children who are uprooted due to unhappy family situations. Multiply that a millionfold and presto—you have God's will and the moral rejuvenation of humankind. The only conclusion to be drawn is, if that is the voice of religion, humankind will be better off without it, as it certainly is better off without war, even a so-called "just" war.

Fortunately, there are traditions which consider *ahiṁsā*, non-killing, non-violence, and mutual helpfulness the first commandment of humanity. These traditions alone deserve the name "religion," if by religion we mean a teaching for the ennoblement of humanity, the realization of its highest potentials and active endeavor to eradicate evil in all forms.

Notes

1. For information on the Bhagavadgītā in general and its interpretations see K. Klostermaier, *A Survey of Hinduism*, Chapter 6, "The Bhagavadgītā."

2. See Duncan M. Derret, "The Concept of Duty in Ancient Indian Jurisprudence," in *The Concept of Duty in South Asia*, 18–65.

3. More detail in K. Klostermaier, "On the Ethical Standards of the Bhagavadgītā," in *Religious Movements in India*, 136–155.

4. All quotations are from J. A. B. van Buitenen, *Rāmānuja on the Bhagavadgītā*. Roman numerals followed by regular numerals refer to chapter and verse of the text of the Bhagavadgītā. Numbers in square brackets [00] refer to page numbers in van Buitenen's work.

5. "The blood of martyrs [is] the seed of Christians." A variation on "The blood of Christians is seed" (Tertullian, *Apology*, 50.13).

Works Cited

Derret, Duncan M. 1979. "The Concept of Duty in Ancient Indian Jurisprudence." In *The Concept of Duty in South Asia*, edited by W. D. O'Flaherty and D. M. Derret. New Delhi: Vikas Publishing House.

Deschner, Karlheinz. 1982. *Ein Jahrhundert Heilsgeschichte. Die Politik der Päpste im Zeitalter der Weltkriege*. Von Leo XIII 1878 bis Pius XI 1939. Köln: Liepenheuer & Witsch.

Klostermaier, K. 1994. *A Survey of Hinduism* (Second edition). Albany, NY: State University of New York Press.

———— 1990. "On the Ethical Standards of the Bhagavadgītā." In *Religious Movements in India*, edited by M. Bardwell Smith. New Delhi: Chanakya.

van Buitenen, J. A. B. 1968. *Rāmānuja on the Bhagavadgītā, A Condensed Rendering of his Gītābhāsya with Copious Notes and an Introduction*. Delhi: Motilal Banarsidass.

Chapter 5

Life, Death and Enlightenment: Buddhist Ethics in a Chinese Context

Albert Welter

Buddhist Ethics in a Chinese Context

Students investigating Chinese Buddhism are confronted with several problems. The most important of these is the dual character of Chinese Buddhism itself. Buddhism was, at least initially, a foreign religion in China. As such, it had to adapt to a foreign cultural setting and espoused native value system. In its earliest phase of intellectual development, China came to be dominated by two indigenous traditions: Confucianism and Taoism. Of these two, Confucianism played the leading role, especially where social and ethical practices were concerned. As Buddhism gained in popularity, it found itself in frequent conflict with native Chinese, i.e., Confucian, ethical concerns. In spite of the common injunctions that ethical systems share, i.e., to do good, be honest, trustworthy, and the like, the basic values of Confucianism and Buddhism placed them at far ends of the ethical spectrum.

It is difficult to characterize the difference between Confucian and Buddhist orientations in a few words. Many Confucian textual sources could be referred to for their ethical content, but in terms of the basic Confucian orientation, the *Great Learning* (*Ta-hsüeh*) can serve as a prime example. The *Great Learning* is a short essay contained in the *Record of Ritual Conduct* (*li-chi*), one of five canonical sources in early Confucianism.[1] Traditionally, these works were thought to have either recorded Confucius' own teachings, or to have been edited by him. The *Great Learning* was later selected by Neo-Confucians (c. 1300) as one of the primary sources for the study of Confucianism.[2] As such, it played a major role in shaping Confucian consciousness.

The *Great Learning* lays out a program of self-cultivation in conjunction with the goals of the state and society. Cultivation of the personal life is the root or foundation for harmony within the family, society, the state, and the world at large. As described in the *Great Learning*, this program of self-cultivation in conjunction with social and state aims is comprised of eight components, each of which is deemed as requisite for fulfilling the one that follows:

1. the investigation of things
2. the extension of knowledge
3. sincerity of the will
4. rectification of the mind
5. cultivation of the personal life
6. regulation of the family
7. ordering the state
8. ensuring peace throughout the world

The first five of these relate specifically to personal cultivation, which "all must regard . . . as the root or foundation" (Chan, *A Source Book in Chinese Philosophy*, 87). The remaining three are matters relating to the fabric of society, the family, the state, and the world at large. Personal cultivation through moral education forms the essential core of the Confucian system. Once this is achieved, it is necessarily applied outwardly, as one's circumstances determine, to family and social responsibilities. The point to be emphasized here is that the basic Confucian orientation is outward, aimed at activities in this world. It is the outward, this-worldly orientation of Confucianism that provides its social and political emphasis.[3] As a result, Confucianism tends to be ambivalent, at best, toward purely spiritual activities, judging spiritual, other-worldly goals as dangerously misdirected and a waste of precious human effort.

Buddhism, on the other hand, aims at release from this world of suffering (*dukkha*), characterized as an endless cycle of birth and death (*samsāra*). The point of human activity is to penetrate the veil of ignorance formed by our illusory sense of permanence. Cultivation based on such insight into the true nature of reality eventually leads to *nirvana*, release from the bounds of created existence and an end to the cycle of rebirth. A convenient contrast to the Confucian program in the *Great Learning* set forth above, is the Buddhist eightfold path of proper conduct, established to lead practitioners to *nirvana*:

1. right understanding
2. right intention

3. right speech
4. right action
5. right livelihood
6. right effort
7. right mindfulness
8. right concentration

According to Buddhist teaching, the first two items relate to the cultivation of wisdom (*prajñâ*), the next three to moral cultivation (*sila*), and the last three to contemplation (*samâdhi*), the three major components of Buddhist cultivation. The contrast with Confucianism is readily apparent. Without knowing the details on how the categories were approached, Confucians would be inclined to concur with the Buddhist emphasis on wisdom and morality as essential areas for personal cultivation. Buddhist meditation practice, however, strikes Confucians as too self-absorbed, too far removed from the tangible world that Confucians tend to accept as real and as the basic realm for positive human interaction. To the Confucians, *nirvana* is too abstract, simply the product of human imagination, to serve as a basis for guiding one's activities. What is worse, devotion to such an other-worldly, spiritual goal will distract one from the social and familial responsibilities which are at the heart of the Confucian view of human nature. From the Buddhist perspective, the same familial and social responsibilities distract one away from the investigation of one's true nature and the discovery that the world we inhabit is fundamentally devoid of any permanent entity (soul or god) to depend on. To the extent that one is absorbed in the affairs of the world, one is liable to misunderstand the basic nature of the circumstances one encounters. Acting on the basis of this misunderstanding will only further enmesh one in the realm of desire. In short, worldly obligations do not encourage dispassion, the prerequisite Buddhist virtue for calming the turbid waters of one's karmic disposition.

The reason for this excursion into the different aims of Confucian and Buddhist thought is because Chinese Buddhism is frequently misunderstood, dismissed as irrelevant and "un-Chinese" by those who assume a monolithic Confucian dominance over everything traditionally Chinese, and reduced to a "perversion" by those who assume that the model of "proper" Buddhism is inextricably Indian in character. By these criteria, Western Christianity could just as readily be rendered as unoriginal, a derivative "bastardization" of Judaism and Greek philosophy. Like Christianity in the West, Chinese Buddhism must be approached as "a system *sui generis*, the result of an independent development which can only be studied and understood in connection with the cultural environment in which this development took place and against the background of the Chinese world view prevailing at the period in question" (Zürcher, *Buddhist Conquest of China*, 1).

The dual character of Chinese Buddhism makes it an especially interesting subject for the study of ethics. Chinese Buddhists operated in a complex world where ethical decisions had to be managed between competing value systems. For example, the decision to enter the Buddhist clergy, the surest way to make progress toward enlightenment, conflicted squarely with the Confucian virtue of filial piety (*hsiao*), respect of children for their parents. As a virtue, filial piety comes close to an "absolute" in Confucian ethics. It includes several dimensions, ranging from obedience to one's parents, support for them in old age, religious rituals honoring family ancestors, and the perpetuation of the family line through the production of male heirs. The decision to leave one's family and enter a Buddhist monastery in pursuit of the ultimate Buddhist goal, *nirvana*, amounts to an abrogation of one's filial duties as prescribed by Confucianism.[4]

In any context, ethical decisions are ultimately made by individuals. By following the choices that individuals make, we can begin to understand what it meant to operate within the world of assumptions that guided the individual's activities. The case I introduce here is not "typical" in the sense that the decisions made were ordinary ones. To the contrary, the example of Yung-ming Yen-shou is noteworthy because he made remarkable decisions under unusual circumstances. Yen-shou emerged from his confrontation with death as a person of integrity. He commanded great respect as a Buddhist leader in his own day. His vast learning won for him a reputation among civil leaders and other Buddhists alike. His writings have continued to provide an excellent model for future generations of East Asian Buddhists down to the present day.

Death and Enlightenment in the Life of Yung-ming Yen-shou

Modern studies of Buddhist ethics have tended to center on Buddhist monastic codes, or rules of discipline (*vinaya*), focusing on the avoidance or prevention of wrong-doing.[5] Only recently have studies appeared which explore ethical practice from the perspective of the motivation of the Buddhist practitioner, especially focusing on moral cultivation (*sila*).[6] The present study is based on the latter approach, looking at moral cultivation and ethical decision in the life of an individual practitioner, Yung-ming Yen-shou (904–975).

What is known of Yen-shou's life is filtered through the interpretation of Buddhist hagiographers. As the requisites for Buddhist practice changed within the Chinese Buddhist community, the life of Yen-shou was enhanced to provide a suitable model.[7] In the present study, I will confine my review of Yen-shou's life to biographies compiled by contemporaries: *Biographies of Eminent Monks compiled in the Sung Dynasty* (*Sung kao-seng chuan*) by Tsan-ning in 988; and *The Transmission of the Lamp,* compiled in the Ching-te era (*Ching-te ch'uan-teng lu*) by Tao-yüan in 1004.[8] These collections are generally devoid of the miraculous and supernatural episodes that play an important role in later records of Yen-shou's life where Yen-shou acquires the persona of a Buddhist saint and cult figure. Even so, we are limited by the information that Yen-shou's bi-ographers chose to record and to some degree by the perspective they adopted.

Little is known of Yen-shou's youth. He was born into a family by the name of Wang in the greater Ch'ien-t'ang area (modern day Hang-chou). By all accounts, he must have followed something of a conventional career path. He undoubtedly received a traditional education in the Confucian classics, and was probably exposed to Buddhist teachings from an early age. At some point in his twenties, he served as a government official in the kingdom of Wu-yüeh. Government service was a mark of success for any male family member. It was the career path of choice among China's traditional elite.

During the tenth century, China had fallen into political and social chaos. The great cosmopolitan era of the T'ang dynasty (619–906) ended when the central government lost control of the military, and regional warlords rose to become masters of independent kingdoms. A period of civil war followed, with warlords competing with each other for power. This is the situation that prevailed in China through much of the tenth century. Along the southeast coast of China, the kingdom of Wu-yüeh (roughly the boundaries of modern day Che-chiang province) was relatively isolated from the war and chaos that plagued the rest of China. Under peaceful conditions and with a prospering economy, Wu-yüeh rulers were able to rebuild civilization and culture in the region. Wu-yüeh borders were strategically important for insulating the kingdom from the chaos that prevailed outside and threatened to engulf it. At the age of twenty-eight, the young Wang (i.e., Yen-shou) was assigned as Garrison Commander in Hua-t'ing, one of the border towns protecting the Wu-yüeh kingdom. At the same time that his career as a military official flourished, he became attracted to the Buddhist teachings of Master Ts'ui-yen. The precise nature of the attraction is not known. We do know, however, that his interest in Buddhism was serious. It lead to the most important decision of his life and the turning point in his career.

In his capacity as Garrison Commander Wang, Yen-shou was in charge of munitions and had considerable financial resources at his disposal. In the context of the times, this was a militarily sensitive and strategically important res-ponsibility. What does a person with sensitive military obligations do when moved by the spirit of Buddhist altruism? Confucian values emphasize the virtues of loyalty in official service to the point where it is paramount. Potential conflicts between filial piety (*hsiao*), respect for one's parents, and loyalty to one's ruler (*ch'ung*) tended to be glossed over in the Confucian tradition by the suggestion that ruler and parent were but two aspects of a continuity: the parent is the ruler of the household as the ruler is the father of his kingdom. Implicit in the attitude of loyalty where military affairs are concerned is the value placed on protecting one's community and state, a civil responsibility upon which the ruler's success depends. In the Chinese context, the failure of a ruler to provide for the peace, prosperity, welfare, and security of his people was deemed a sign of Heaven's displeasure. Prolonged failings on the part of a ruler were interpreted as certain demise. According to the Confucian justification for dynastic change, Heaven, the concept for divine will that ensures cosmic harmony, revokes a ruler's mandate (*t'ien-ming*) under such circumstances and places it in the hands of someone more worthy. The ability to preserve harmony on earth, in society and even in the natural order, was deemed a reflection of the moral character of the ruler himself. Given these criteria, a failed ruler was always considered lacking in moral virtue.

Garrison Commander Wang, a person of official position, served as a representative of his ruler. The ruler depended on the services of people like Commander Wang to fulfill the important duties of state and society that fell under his purview. Wang's failure threatened the carefully constructed security and prosperity that the citizens of Wu-yüeh enjoyed. Why Commander Wang chose to ignore the time-honored demands of loyalty of military subordinates to their superiors is difficult to fathom. What we do know is that he was moved by Buddhist compassion, and that he chose to exercise his compassion by illegally appropriating funds under his command to buy living creatures and set them free.[9] Buying living creatures, usually caged birds or fish, had become a customary practice in China. Some temples made profits by keeping such items on hand, so that Buddhist aspirants could readily express their compassion, believing to receive spiritual rewards or merit in return. When Commander Wang chose to relieve the suffering of these living beings, however, his motivation went far beyond the ordinary, prescribed practice for earning merit.

Commander Wang's actions can only be described as those of someone for whom the world he has lived in, the principles he has lived by, no longer make sense. The actions of a person, committed to a sense of values, who begins to contradict the principles he has been committed to in an apparently self-destructive way, are the actions of someone in the process of radical transformation. Nowhere does Yen-shou in his writings address his motivation for this action directly. Implicit in his actions, however, is a profound sense of frustration with the world around him, part of a seemingly futile search for temporal peace and order where experience shows how military success and economic prosperity are fleeting, where chaos and suffering are the order of the day. Emerging in Commander Wang is a sense that the true solution, to Wu-yüeh's problems, to China's problems, to the problems of human existence, is not simply an affirmation or imposition of social and political order. The real solution is coming to terms with human nature. This demands a radical transformation of the human personality. Only Buddhism, according to Commander Wang, can effect such a transformation. When Commander Wang released the living creatures, he recognized their imprisonment as his own. As a Buddhist, it was easy for him to recognize in them an existence only marginally different from his own. Such creatures also possessed a spirit and were caught in the same cycle of *samsāra* as he himself. Their release symbolized his own longing to be free of the conventions that bound him to futile actions that supported a military establishment ultimately committed to destroying life (or at preserving some lives at the expense of others) rather than saving it.

The Buddhist principles that Commander Wang was devoted to demanded allegiance to a higher truth. Confucian virtues only provided harmony within the limited context of the human social order. Buddhist teachings demanded that one see beyond such a narrow perspective, bound to the realities of this world and one's present lifespan, and acknowledge the interconnectedness between oneself and all created existence. On the basis of this realization, one must endeavor to alleviate the suffering of all created beings. This is the vow of the *bodhisattva*, the model Buddhist practitioner according to the Mahayana tradition.

Commander Wang's own release from death would prove to be more difficult than that of the creatures he had set free. Under civil law, Wang was at best an unrepentant thief and disloyal official. Under the sensitive military circumstances, his actions could be construed as treasonous, jeopardizing the security of the entire region. Under no circumstances could Commander Wang's crime be taken lightly. The punishment had to reflect the seriousness of the infraction and act as a deterrence to others. Commander Wang was sentenced to death. Following a long tradition in China of conscientious objectors and others who wanted to avoid military conscription, Commander Wang took refuge in a Buddhist monastery, leaving his wife and child,[10] becoming a student of Master Ts'ui-yen, and taking the Buddhist name Yen-shou ("Prolonger of Life").

Throughout history, Chinese governments frequently criticized Buddhism for harboring criminals, including men who entered the Buddhist clergy to escape military conscription. By law, Buddhist monasteries were tax exempt, self-governing bodies over which civil law had little jurisdiction. Whether or not

Buddhist monasteries were really the hotbeds of criminal, licentious activity that Confucian critics often suggested is highly doubtful. What Buddhist monasteries did represent, was an alternate institutional structure that competed with the central government for resources and influence. It also suggested a different ideological orientation toward the world, one that conflicted with the code of loyalty and social responsibility that the state endorsed. Buddhist monasteries offered an escape from the onerous nexus of social responsibility, a refuge where individuals could pursue spiritual goals free of vexing social concerns.

Roughly a century before this incident involving Yen-shou took place, the Chinese government mounted a comprehensive campaign to curb the influence of Buddhism in Chinese society. Temples and monasteries were closed. Only a few temples in any given region were allowed to remain open, under government jurisdiction. Buddhist lands and amassed wealth were returned to government control. Strict guidelines were enacted to determine who could legitimately join the Buddhist clergy. Many of the harshest measures of the purge were either rescinded or never fully enacted, so that the impact was not as severe as it might have been. The overall direction, however, was clear. Governments would exert increasing control over the Buddhist presence in China. This marked the beginning of the end of Buddhist independence.[11] This meant Yen-shou could not avoid criminal prosecution, even given his newly acquired status as a member of the Buddhist clergy. The death sentence was not rescinded.

Fortunately for Yen-shou, however, the rulers of Wu-yüeh, the Ch'ien family, were devout supporters of Buddhism. They looked to the "golden age" of Buddhism in China, the T'ang dynasty, for their model. Economic prosperity in Wu-yüeh meant that the rulers had ample resources to rebuild their kingdom. Much of their effort aimed at rebuilding Buddhist temples, shrines, and monasteries. They conceived Buddhism as the central ideology of their kingdom, and Buddhist monks occupied important roles in state and local affairs. The kingdom of Wu-yüeh was a Buddhist kingdom; its rulers consciously emulated the famed Indian Buddhist monarch Ashoka, who served as the model for Buddhist secular rulers. Building activities transformed Wu-yüeh into the most important Buddhist center in China within the span of a few decades.

Rather than ruthlessly condemn Yen-shou as a criminal, the Wu-yüeh ruler sent an emissary to observe Yen-shou's reaction when the death sentence was announced. If Yen-shou expressed grief, or reacted emotionally in any way, the emissary was instructed, this should be interpreted that Yen-shou had not really transcended the cares of this world and the sentence should be carried out. If, however, Yen-shou was dispassionate and calmly accepted his fate, this should be taken as a sign of true Buddhist devotion, and Yen-shou should be granted permission to enter the Buddhist clergy and assume the life of a monk. According to reports, Yen-shou confronted death calmly. He showed no emotion and did not object when the sentence was announced. Like the animals that Yen-shou had released, Yen-shou himself was granted freedom by the ruler. Rather than a strict sense of justice, the prevailing mode for arriving at moral decisions was the exercise of Buddhist compassion. It was compassion, rather than a sense of duty or obligation to one's task, that compelled Yen-shou to break his worldly oath in service of a higher truth. It was the same sense of compassion that compelled the ruler to rescind Yen-shou's sentence. It is not unusual in the history of religions to find religious figures invoking "the spirit" as superior to human law. It is unusual to find secular rulers who do so. In East Asian circles, a distinction was made between *wang-fa* (Japanese *ôhô*) and *fo-fa* (Japanese *buppô*), literally "the king's law" and "the Buddha's law." Typically, even rulers who supported Buddhism were careful to mark the appropriate jurisdiction of each, so that Buddhist teaching did not interfere in the exercise of secular affairs.

Through this episode, Yen-shou won a reputation as a charismatic religious figure. His devotion to Buddhism, rooted in Buddhist compassion, allowed him to "cheat death," as if he already had a foothold on immortality. In spite of the subtleties of Buddhist teachings regarding the ultimate falsity of such conceptions as an individual "soul" (*atman*) or "immortality," the Chinese common people had long accepted the Buddhist religion on precisely these grounds. Yen-shou, in their eyes, became a living embodiment of this possibility.

Yen-shou went on to study Buddhism under the leading masters of the region. In 952, he took up residence at a temple on Mt. Hsüeh-tou and began attracting students. In 960, on the strength of his scholasticism, Yen-shou was invited by Wu-yüeh rulers to become the abbot of one of the regions most prestigious temples, the Ling-yin Temple. The following year, he was reassigned to the Yung-ming Temple, a Buddhist temple constructed by Wu-yüeh rulers as a crowning monument to the Wu-yüeh Buddhist revival. Over the next fifteen years, Yen-shou presided over Wu-yüeh Buddhism as its leading spokesperson. Monks from throughout China flocked to Wu-yüeh to study with Yen-shou. He is reported to have had 1,700 students. The king of Korea sent gifts honoring Yen-shou, beseeching him to accept a contingent of Korean Buddhist monks as students. After Yen-shou's death, his reputation as a cult figure among Chinese Buddhists continued to the extent that his tomb became a pilgrimage site for those seeking rebirth in the Pure Land. His writings became a major source from which future students studied Buddhism in Japan and Korea, as well as China.

In conclusion, I would like to point to two cases where Yen-shou's writings are connected to his own life experience. The first is his defense of self-sacrifice as an expression of one's highest realization. The second is his appropriation of Confucian ethics into a Buddhist framework.

Enlightenment Through Death: In Defense of Self-Sacrifice

Through personal experience, Yen-shou understood how death could be faced calmly and dispassionately. Rather than a nihilistic urge or a fatalistic resignation, Yen-shou saw one's ability to confront death in positive terms as denying the power that death has over one. In his writings, Yen-shou went even further to suggest that one could legitimately sacrifice one's own life. Yen-shou argued that not only could such actions be deemed morally justifiable, they could even constitute expressions of enlightenment itself.

Within the Buddhist tradition, self-sacrifice is treated with a high degree of ambiguity. The taking of life, including one's own, is roundly condemned as a serious offense according to the *vinaya* rules.[12] In other circumstances, however, the Buddhist tradition takes a more tolerant attitude toward the practice. The Mahayana tradition, for example, positively affirmed the practice of self-immolation in the *Lotus Sutra*.[13] Mahayana Buddhists, as a result, speak positively of *bodhisattvas* offering their lives to assist others. All three of the *Biographies of Eminent Monks* collections, a kind of "Lives of Buddhist Saints in China," contain categories for monks who achieved their status through self-sacrifice. In response to obvious criticism for including them, the authors of each collection concur that although self-sacrifice is wrong from the viewpoint of the monastic rules which clearly forbid it, it is to be admired if one takes into account the attitude and courage of the doer.[14] In his writings, Yen-shou staunchly defended the practice.

> When one relinquishes one's physical body, terminating one's life in order to reciprocate the kindness of the Dharma, one is in tacit agreement with the greater vehicle and in deep accord with true Buddhist teaching. (*Taishô shinshû daizôkyô*, vol. 48.969b)

For Yen-shou, relinquishing one's physical body is justifiable as an act of almsgiving, one of six practices to be perfected (*pâramitâ*) in the attainment of bodhisattva virtues. According to Yen-shou there are two kinds of almsgiving: ordinary outward almsgiving that is a traditional mainstay of monastic life, and inward almsgiving—the sacrifice of one's entire self as an expression of enlightenment. The crucial criteria for determining the validity of self-sacrifice rests in the attitude and understanding of the person when the act is committed.

According to Yen-shou, if such acts are the result of sincerity and devotion to Buddhism and based on illuminating insight, they serve as means to exchange mortal existence for an immortal one, an end to *samsāra* and the occasion for great liberation (*Taishô shinshû daizôkyô*, vol. 48.972c).

In terms of the larger body of Yen-shou's thought, such acts constitute an actualization of enlightenment. Rather than a theoretical understanding, enlightenment for Yen-shou was something that had to be concretely demonstrated through one's practices. It was important for Yen-shou that enlightenment had to be practiced with the body, not just conceived with the mind. Under proper circumstances, the act of self-sacrifice may serve as a perfect demonst⌐ .ion oi one's enlightened nature.

Yen-shou relied on a common Buddhist framework for his position, viewing self-sacrifice in terms of the interplay between *prajñâ*-wisdom and skillful means (*upâya*). Without skillful means to express one's wisdom, one is reduced to a state of non-activity, or passivity. Without wisdom to guide one's activities, one becomes absorbed in the realm of illusions, mistaking it as real. Only when *prajñâ*-wisdom and skillful means are acknowledged as uniform extensions of each other and not as a duality will the enlightened nature of reality be revealed (*Taishô shinshû daizôkyô*, vol. 48.972a).

Chinese Ethics in a Buddhist Context

Throughout his life, Yen-shou acknowledged the pluralistic nature of the society around him. His own transformation from official to monk contrasted sharply with rising anti-Buddhist attitudes in China. Over a century earlier, the Confucian official Han Yü struck out at the pervasive Buddhist presence in China, characterizing it as a blight on China's Confucian character. He called on the emperor to purge China of Buddhism on the bases that it was un-Chinese ("no more than a cult of the barbarian peoples"), subversive of public morality ("our old ways [will] be corrupted, our customs violated"), and superstitious ("How . . . could [the Buddha's] rotten bones . . . be rightly admitted to the palace [for worship]?").[15]

Yen-shou's response to the Confucian revival and to Confucian attacks on Buddhism was conciliatory. As his own career showed, Yen-shou had no doubt regarding the superiority of Buddhist teaching over Confucianism. In his writings, however, he did grant Confucian teachings a viable, if subordinate place. He acknowledged Confucians as *bodhisattvas* who through their moral teachings and insights paved the way for Buddhism in China.

Confucius . . . practiced loyalty (*chung*) and established filial piety (*hsiao*). He elucidated virtue (*te*), and imparted humaneness (*jen*). But he only spread good in the world, and was not able to liberate the spirit by abandoning verbal explanations. As a result, his was not a great awakening. (*Taishô shinshû daizôkyô*, vol. 48.987c)

However beneficial the practice of Confucian virtues may be, such practices are ultimately lacking for the reasons suggested above. Confucian virtues may complement practices based on Buddhist insight, but they can never serve as a substitute for them, much less as their replacement.

In this way, Yen-shou offered a typically Buddhist response to the problem of ethical pluralism in the Chinese context. Confucian morality was encouraged as supportive of family and social interests. It encouraged people to be good citizens and act decently toward one another. It was not to be taken as the ultimate standard for behavior, however, as it was based on a limited understanding of this world and the nature of created existence.

Yen-shou experienced personal transformation during the chaotic times of tenth century China, a period marked by civil conflict and social upheaval. This transformation became the strength from which Yen-shou drew, the seed of a new perception from which to understand the world. In important respects, the ethical situation Yen-shou faced is not unlike our own. Broadly speaking, we too are faced with vastly different criteria for making ethical decisions. The humanistic tradition which informs much of what we call secular liberalism assumes a human-centered universe limited to the sense-based observations of the external world. We who accept this, struggle for meaning within the parameters that these limitations allow. What exists beyond this we may speculate on and muse over, but never know with certainty. The extent to which these speculations and musings affect our personal decisions and behavior is largely a private matter to which we are entitled so long as it does not transgress the rules of the secular order. Our other choice, broadly speaking, is to accept some version of a traditionally religious perspective, acknowledging our own human existence not as the measure of our knowledge, but as a part of a larger reality. This reality cannot be proven under the criteria of modern science, but can only be intuited through the shadowy intervals of human experience. Like Yen-shou, we may affirm one as more true than the other, but confronted with the reality of both in our daily lives, we manage some kind of compromise between them. This compromise becomes the basis for the ethical decisions from which our actions arise.

Notes

1. The five canonical sources in early Confucianism were *The Book of Documents* (*shu-ching*), *The Book of Poetry* (*shih-ching*), *Record of Ritual Conduct* (*li-chi*), *Spring and Autumn Annals* (*ch'un-ch'iu*), and *The Book of Changes* (*i-ching*).

2. Along with the *Great Learning*, the "classics" of Neo-Confucianism include the *Analects* (*Lun-yü*) of Confucius, the *Mencius* (*Meng-tzu*), and the *Doctrine of the Mean* (*Ch'ung-yung*).

3. My characterization of Confucianism as "this worldly" and Buddhism as "other worldly" follows Max Weber, "The Social Psychology of the World Religions," in *Max Weber: Essays in Sociology*, 267–301.

4. For a comprehensive discussion of how Chinese Buddhists accommodated Confucian filial demands, see Kenneth K. S. Ch'en, *The Chinese Transformation of Buddhism*, chapter two, "Ethical Life," 14–64.

5. See Charles S. Prebish, *A Survey of Vinaya Literature*.

6. A good example is that of David W. Chappell, "Searching for a Mahâyâna Social Ethic," *Journal of Religious Ethics* 1996: 351–375— a study that approaches Buddhist ethics from the Mahâyâna motivation of "saving all beings."

7. On the development of Yen-shou's biographical image see Albert Welter, *The Meaning of Myriad Good Deeds*; Part II, "The Life of Yung-ming Yen-shou: the Making of a Ch'an and Pure Land Patriarch," 37–108; and "The Contextual Study of Buddhist Biographies: The Example of Yung-ming Yen-shou (904–975),"in *Monks and Magicians: Religious Biographies in Asia*, 247–268.

8. Both collections are included in the modern Japanese edition of the Chinese Buddhist Canon, *Taishô shinshû daizôkyô* (Tokyo, 1924–1934), vol. 50.887a–b and vol. 51.421c–422a.

9. There is some uncertainty here due to the fact that it is only in later sources that the full version of this episode is recounted. Earliest sources tend to gloss over it, the reasons for which are explored in my other writings on Yen-shou cited above. Although the details remain hazy, my conclusion is that some such episode did in fact occur.

10. This is mentioned in only one source, the earliest biography compiled by Tsan-ning in the *Sung kao-seng chuan*. It is an obvious parallel with the life of the Buddha, and may have been included for that reason. It may have been omitted in later sources because of its offensiveness to Chinese sensibilities regarding the inviolability of the family.

11. In Chinese history, this period is known as the Hui-ch'ang suppression (c.840–845), after the reign title of the current Chinese emperor. Those interested in investigating this further may wish to consult Kenneth Ch'en, *Buddhism in China: A Historical Survey*, 226–233.

12. One of the *pârâjika* rules, violation of which demand permanent expulsion from the Buddhist order, states: "If a monk should intentionally take the life of a human being or of one

like a human being, with his own hand, or with a knife, or by having him assassinated, then he has fallen into an offence which deserves expulsion. And this applies also to a monk who incites others to self-destruction, and who speaks to them in praise of death, with words such as, 'O man, what is the use to you of this miserable life? It is better for you to die than be alive!'" (Edward Conze, *Buddhist Scriptures*, 74).

13. A popular model for self-immolation practice for Mahayana practitioners was provided by the chapter of the *Lotus Sutra* entitled "The Former Affairs of the Bodhisattva Medicine King (Sanskrit, Bhaisajyarâja)." See, for example, Burton Watson, *The Lotus Sutra*, 280–289).

14. The Chinese perspective on self-immolation is presented through a study of the three *Biographies of Eminent Monks* collections by Jan Yün-hua, "Buddhist Self-Immolation in Medieval China," *History of Religions*, 243–265.

15. Quotes in parenthesis are from Han Yü's "Memorial on the Bone of the Buddha,"in *Sources of Chinese Tradition*, vol. 1, 372–374.

Works Cited

Chan, Wing-tsit, comp. and trans. 1963. *A Source Book in Chinese Philosophy.* Princeton: Princeton University Press.

Chappell, David W. 1996. "Searching for a Mahâyâna Social Ethic." *Journal of Religious Ethics*, vol. 24, no. 2: 351–375.

Ch'en, Kenneth K. S. 1973. *The Chinese Transformation of Buddhism.* Princeton: Princeton University Press.

———. 1964. *Buddhism in China: A Historical Survey.* Princeton: Princeton University Press.

Chinese Buddhist Canon. 1924–1934. *Taishô shinshû daizôkyô.* Edited by Takakusu Junjiro and Watanabe Kaikyoku. Tokyo: Taisho issaikyo kankokai.

Conze, Edward. 1959. *Buddhist Scriptures: A Bibliography.* London: Penguin Books.

Granoff, Phyllis, and Koichi Shinohara, eds. 1988. *Monks and Magicians: Religious Biographies in Asia.* Oakville, ON: Mosaic Press.

Prebish, Charles S. 1994. *A Survey of Vinaya Literature.* Taipei: Jin Luen Publishing House.

Watson, Burton, trans. 1993. *The Lotus Sutra.* New York: Columbia University Press.

Weber, Max. 1946. "The Social Psychology of the World Religions." In *Max Weber: Essays in Sociology*, edited and translated by H. H. Gerth and C. Wright Mills. New York: Oxford University Press.

Welter, Albert. 1993. *The Meaning of Myriad Good Deeds*: A Study of Yung-ming Yen-shou and the Wan-shan t'ung-kuei chi. New York: Peter Lang.

Yü, Han. 1960. "Memorial on the Bone of the Buddha," in *Sources of Chinese Tradition*, edited by William Theodore de Bary, *Sources of Chinese Tradition*. Vol. 1. New York: Columbia University Press, 372–374.

Yün-hua, Jan. 1965. "Buddhist Self-Immolation in Medieval China," *History of Religions* 4: 243–265.

Zürcher, E. 1972. *The Buddhist Conquest of China: The Spread and Adaptation of Buddhism in Early Medieval China.* Leiden: E. J. Brill.

Chapter 6

Revisioning Judaism:
Mordecai Kaplan's Ethics of Immanence

Neal Rose

Jerusalem, winter of 1979-80. It was a cold Friday morning, *erev shabbat*. I and a close friend were standing at the door of the retirement home of the then almost hundred year old Jewish humanistic philosopher and theologian Professor Mordecai Kaplan (1881–1983). My companion, a long time student and associate of Kaplan's, had secured an interview for me with Kaplan.

The philosopher sat in an oversized chair surrounded by his journals. After a brief introduction and general discussion about my research, our mutual friend informed Professor Kaplan that I had a question about his work: "Neal Rose wants to know what you regard as your most important singular work." Kaplan, without hesitation, responded: "Mordecai Kaplan's most important work is *The Meaning of God in Modern Jewish Religion* because in it . . . ." At this point his voice became almost inaudible. Yet, I thought he was saying: "because in it Mordecai Kaplan actually carried out the reconstruction of Jewish religion in the context of modern religious humanism."

Confirmed! My theory for years had been that *The Meaning of God in Modern Jewish Religion*, among all of Kaplan's many works, is the intellectual laboratory for his revisioning of Jewish religion. In his long literary and communal career, Kaplan produced philosophical, theological, liturgical and artistic works. In *Meaning*, however, he attempted to synthesize traditional Jewish religion with modernity. What is found in *Meaning* is not a modernistic apologia for traditional Rabbinic Judaism but an altogether new version of Jewish religion. That the book's title does not contain the term "Judaism" is quite telling: Kaplan wants to depict a version of "Jewish religion" which is quite different from "Judaism," as understood through the traditional Rabbinic world view. In this essay, I will attempt to outline Kaplan's version of "Jewish religion" and to compare it, when helpful, to the Judaism of the traditional, Rabbinic world view. In particular, I will attempt to explicate the life ethics inherent in Kaplan's idea of God and of Jewish religion. The key to this life ethics, and to Kaplan's Jewish religion, is what Israeli philosopher Yirmiyahu Yovel calls "the philosophy of immanence."

Rabbinic Supernaturalism

What is traditional or Rabbinic Judaism? And what about it, in Kaplan's opinion, requires revisioning or reinterpretation?

While many non-Jews, particularly Christians, equate Judaism with the Bible, or with what Christians call the Old Testament, this is an historically inadequate definition. For Judaism, although a religion of the Bible, is also based on extra-Biblical books. To put it another way and in shorthand terms, Judaism is a religion of the Bible as read or interpreted by ancient Jewish scholars who lived hundreds of years after the Biblical period. These scholars, known as teachers or Rabbis, adopted a unique hermeneutics that produced, in turn, a unique Jewish life style that they called the holy "way" or *halachah*. The teachings of these Rabbis (second to seventh century) are collected into a voluminous and composite work know as the Talmud. The religion that emerged from this Talmudic base is known as Rabbinic Judaism. In the late twentieth century, it is also called Orthodox Judaism; the closest contemporary approximation to ancient Talmudic or Rabbinic Judaism.

Modern-day orthodox Jews believe that the ancient Rabbis were empowered by God to interpret the Bible. They further claim that only the Rabbis and their spiritual heirs have the authority to continue to interpret the will of God found in the Torah, the Bible, and in codes of Jewish law. This claim is not new: ancient Rabbis also believed it. Contemporary Orthodox Jews, like the Rabbis, see the Jews as a "chosen people" with a unique relationship to God. Such orthodoxy is not found only in Judaism: Islam and Christianity, also religions of the Bible, have orthodox forms that have produced similar historical claims to uniqueness and exclusive interpretive authority.

What are the major beliefs of Rabbinic Judaism? In the first place, the Rabbinic tradition understands God as a personal Being who created, and continues to recreate, the world. This personal God reveals His teachings to the world at large primarily through the people of Israel. The record of God's revelation is found in the Torah, the so-called Old Testament. God has guided, and continues to guide, and when necessary to intervene in, the affairs of the world. Eventually, God will bring an end to the evil and corruption in the world through his human agent, known as the Messiah. In the Rabbinic tradition, God is understood to reward good and to punish evil, both in this world and in the next, the world we enter after death. Rabbinic Judaism sees this world as a passageway to the next. In this world, all people must submit to the demands, or commands (*mitzvot*), of God. The *mitzvot* consist of a basic morality incumbent upon all people, Jews and non-Jews, as well as an additional *mitzvot* applicable to Jews only. These additional *mitzvot*, many of a ritualistic nature, constitute the *halachah*, or traditional Jewish life style.

The *luach*, the Sacred Calendar of Judaism, is at the center of this life style. The *luach* includes a number of holy days, festivals and fasts: *Sabbath*, a weekly holiday that begins each Friday at sunset and concludes after sunset on Saturday night; *Passover*, a festival of early Spring; *Shavuot*, a late Spring festival; *Sukkot*, a celebration held in late Fall; and *Rosh Hashannah* and *Yom Kippur*, holy days of early Fall. Before we can appreciate Kaplan's heterodox approach to Jewish religion and ethics, we need to discuss the way in which Jewish orthodox understanding of the *luach* is rooted in supernaturalism and notions of the miraculous. For instance, traditional Judaism believes that Passover commemorates the literal Exodus of the Israelites from Egypt, an event accomplished by divine intervention and many supernatural miracles. The Passover story of the Exodus is told through the use of symbols such as lamb and leavened bread. But in Rabbinic orthodoxy, the story of this and other festivals is told in ways that emphasize the miraculous. Rabbinic interpretations of Passover and other Jewish festivals form a master-myth at the core of orthodox theology and ritual. Rabbinic versions of the *luach* emphasize that:

• *God* is a personal being who is the Creator and source of reality. This God is aware of the world and all its doings. He reveals His presence and will to those who live in the world.

• *Torah* is the definitive revelation of God's will. Rabbis of the Talmud best understood revelation, and only their spiritual heirs have the authority to apply the Rabbinic method.

• *Israel* is chosen. While God's Revelation is given to all, it is specifically directed to the people of Israel. They have been chosen to represent and give witness to God's presence in the world.

Kaplan retains the terms God, Torah, and Israel, but he rejects the supernaturalism of orthodoxy, and of orthodox *luach* myth and ritual, because he feels that supernaturalism is untenable in our scientifically-oriented age. Kaplan also dismisses the idea that any religion or group is chosen by God. He prefers to think that the nature of religious uniqueness is the product of historical and cultural conditioning. Interestingly, he is among the first of modern Jewish thinkers to reject sexism in religion and to advocate gender equality. *The Meaning of God in Modern Jewish Religion* is Kaplan's attempt to revision Jewish religion by way of reinterpreting the *luach*. This reinterpretation does away with supernaturalism in favor of a philosophy, and a life ethics, of immanence.

From Spinoza to Kaplan

Yirmiyahu Yovel speaks of Baruch Spinoza (1632–1677) as "the first philosopher of immanence" (Yovel, *Spinoza and Other Heretics*, 169). It seems to me that Kaplan is the first modern Jewish theologian of immanence. What binds Spinoza to Kaplan is the total disavowal they share of supernaturalism and of transcendental explanations of all aspects of life. Both insist that all aspects of reality, including Jewish history and religion, be understood in terms of *immanent* or *inherent this-worldly principles*. What radically distinguishes the two, however, is their attitude to Jews and Jewish tradition. Having disposed of classical Western transcendentalism, especially the transcendentalism of Judaism, Spinoza went on to construct a world view which was supposed to provide a new map of reality and a new path to this-worldly salvation for all people. But as Ben-Ami Scharfstein points out, Spinoza's attitude was hypercritical, if not hateful, toward Jews and Judaism, "more unfavorable than the facts made necessary" (Scharfstein, *Philosophers and Their Lives*, 152). Spinoza was excommunicated from the Jewish community of Amsterdam in 1656, after which he lived in a kind of cultural no-man's land.

By contrast, Kaplan put his philosophy of immanence in service of the Jewish people. Like Spinoza, Kaplan used philosophy of immanence to reconstruct Rabbinic Judaism, but at the same time, Kaplan drew from his philosophy of immanence to construct a new version of Jewish religion. Kaplan thought of philosophy of immanence as a general, or universal, theory which is applicable to all aspects of human culture, especially to religion. For example, he made it abundantly clear that his sociology of religion is applicable to all religions. Similarly, he presented his theory of historiography as universal, and he strongly endorsed modern secular histories of the Jewish people. "If they had not secularized the story of the Jewish past by subjecting it to the laws of historical cause and effect, the Jewish people might have ceased to be a reality and would have evaporated into myth," Kaplan contends (Kaplan, *Not So Random Thoughts*,

292). This endorsement of secularization is part of Kaplan's immanentist critique of Jewish history and culture. It belongs together with his critique of the *sancta*, the symbols, myths, and rituals of Jewish tradition. Through his critique, Kaplan attempts to construct a new version of Jewish religion and ethics.

In *Meaning*, this religious ethics builds on the structure of the Sabbath and the major Jewish holidays. Indeed, Kaplan's book is structured around Jewish holidays. The opening chapter discredits existing interpretations of Judaism, largely because they do not fit the paradigm of immanence, yet the succeeding chapters, laid out according to the traditional Jewish calendar (the Sabbath, *Rosh Hashannah*, the New Year, *Yom Kippur*, the Day of Atonement, etc.) return to and recast the Jewish tradition being critiqued. Each chapter relates to an aspect of God, understood not as person, but as immanent power or energy. As a humanist, Kaplan speaks of God/Godhood as the Power That Makes For Salvation, that makes for the enhancement of human life. This is the meaning of the Sabbath, for Kaplan: its rituals, myths and symbols, point to God as the power or energy that makes for human salvation. Similarly, *Rosh Hashannah*, through its *sancta*, highlights God as the energy that makes for social regeneration. For Kaplan, the ethical impulse comes from the connection people make with this power or energy that flows through the world. Kaplan's God-idea is a process one, and it follows for him that ethics, as the means to "salvation," entails moving with the process or power that is immanent in the world.

The close relationship that exists for Kaplan between process theology and ethics leads him to speak of the "soterical God-idea." By this, Kaplan means a way of talking about God that heightens our awareness of the forces or powers that make for this-worldly salvation. Kaplan asks whether his "soterical God-idea" implies a God that can be worshiped. He answers in the affirmative, although he is careful to define the role of worship: the purpose of worship and prayer, says Kaplan, is to produce awareness. He turns here to philosopher/psychologist William James' comments about prayer as the "vital act by which the entire mind seeks to save itself by clinging to the principle from which it draws life" (Kaplan, *The Future of the American Jew*, 183–84). In other words, prayer is a form of consciousness-raising about the "Godly" powers within the outer world as well as the inner world of self, powers that lead to enhancement of life on this earth.

The significance of the soterical God-idea is perhaps best seen in Kaplan's concern for educating the young. Kaplan's pedagogical theory begins not with the inculcation of tradition but with making children aware of God's reality in the world. Kaplan advocates the need to make children conscious of the creativity and growth taking place all around them. Perhaps even more urgent is the need to ensure that children experience their own growth and development: "There can hardly be a more real and more God-revealing experience in the inner life of a child than that of growth" (*Future of the American Jew*, 186). Once made aware of their growth, Jewish children can be taught their traditions in the context of what Kaplan calls the soterical imperative, the need to connect with the powers of the immanent God.

On the positive side, Kaplan defines the immanent God as "the creative life of the universe" (*Meaning of God*, 76). God can be said to be "the sum of the animating, organizing forces and relationships which are forever making a cosmos out of chaos" (76). The word "forever" here suggests finitude: incompleteness and fragmentation. Kaplan dismisses the transcendental notion of "God as infinite and perfect in His omniscience and omnipotence." Rather, he writes that "God does not have to mean to us an absolute being who has planned and decreed every twinge of pain, every act of cruelty, every humanism" (76). Kaplan uses the term "God," but his use of the term does not do away with the radical finitude of the universe, of a world that has not yet "reached finality, but is continually being renewed by God and in need of improvement by men" (76). Nor does Kaplan's term "God" imply a transcendental other-worldly perfect being. Indeed, it was Kaplan's dedication to naturalism that led him to write *Judaism Without Supernaturalism* (1958). And it is from the point of view of this vision of immanence that Kaplan, in *Meaning*, tries to read, or as he puts it, to "reevaluate," Jewish sacred literature. Revelation, in traditional Judaism, is seen as a once-and-for-all-time event. Revelation, for Kaplan, keeps happening throughout history. Revelation and redemption are, and will always remain, incomplete: the dance of cosmos/chaos will go on forever.[1]

Those who knew Kaplan agree that his life experience led him directly and increasingly to this vision of immanence. Influenced by the pragmatism of such American thinkers as William James, John Dewey and C. S. Pierce, Kaplan was convinced that human experience, not dogmatic tradition, is the basis of human salvation and human ethics. The strong emphasis on experience is seen early on in *Meaning*, where Kaplan criticizes the early twentieth century liberal Jewish theologian Kaufman Kohler for his over intellectualization of Judaism. Kaplan refers to Kohler's work as "a rehash, not even warmed over, of medieval verbalism" (*Meaning of God*, 16). Worst of all, Kaplan maintains, this verbalism is divorced from facts and realities humans know and experience in everyday life.[2] Kaplan sees traditional Rabbinic Judaism overall as authoritarian and hierarchical and removed from lived experience. His commitment to immanence leads to his rejection of all perceived authoritarian elements of tradition. Emanuel Goldsmith sums this point up when he says that Kaplan's rejection "of belief in God as a supernatural being" is not isolated but includes the rejection of authoritarianism and any attempt to anchor the validation of authority in the supernatural. Goldsmith points out that Kaplan also rejects "the supernatural people-idea commonly known as chosenness and the supernatural revelation-idea known as *Torah min hashamayim*" (Goldsmith, *Dynamic Judaism*, 19). Having dismissed traditional supernaturalism and salvationism, Kaplan substitutes for them his "axiom of experience" as salvific, and his life ethics also founded on experience, rather than on the authority of the Rabbinic past.

Introducing Kaplan's Life Ethics

For Kaplan, ethics defines the norms that are needed for this-worldly salvation. The search for this-worldly salvation requires that we accept it as true that "reality is so constituted as to endorse and guarantee the realization in man of that which is a greatest value to him" (*Meaning of God*, 29). In believing this, Kaplan says, "we have faith in God" (29), where God is understood as the Power that makes for social regeneration, regeneration of human nature, cooperation, freedom, and righteousness. In other words, there is a direct correlation for Kaplan between human values and cosmic energies. This, it seems to me, might be called Kaplan's "principle of correlation," a term that would indicate how, for Kaplan, basic principles of ethics are not merely human ideas but parallels to cosmic forces that are operative throughout the universe. It is Kaplan's "principle of correlation" that breaks down the traditional division between objectivity and subjectivity, between the outer world of nature and the inner world of human thought and ethical action. Kaplan, many years after *Meaning*, still sums all of this up as the soterical God-idea.[3]

Most ethical theories ask a number of related questions about human beings: 1) What is human? 2) What is the moral problem for humans? 3) What solution to this problem is available to humans? In answer to the first question, What is human?, it needs for our purposes to be said that Kaplan understands the human person to be a self-actualizing being who lives in the context of a larger social grouping. In answer to the second question, What is the moral problem for humans?, Kaplan points out that often a person is hindered in his or her development either because of personal faults and/or due to problems generated by society. In answer to the third question, What solution to the problem is available for humans?, Kaplan asserts his belief that the universe is geared to human self-actualization, and that it is therefore necessary for people to become aware of those forces which make for their salvation. This awareness cannot be gained alone but requires the creation of a growth-promoting culture.

On the basis of this, we should not be surprised to find that Kaplan's life ethics combines an individual with a communitarian perspective. In his discussion of the closing Fall holiday *Shemini Azeret*, for instance, Kaplan talks about the absolute need of people, individually and communally, to experience the presence of God. God, he writes, is more than an idea. God "must be felt as a presence, if we want not only to know about God but to know God" (*Meaning of God*, 244). He goes on to say that "religious souls have never been satisfied with an awareness of God merely as an intellectual concept." What do they crave? They crave the immediate experience of God. It is this experience which, Kaplan says, compels "our adoration and worship." It is this experiential component that converts religious teachings "from theology to religion." Without this experience, he says, we have humanism and not religion. And only with this experience do we have people feeling that their "ethical aspirations are part of the cosmic urge." Further, people need to gain, through experience, a sensed reality of the "inner harmony between human nature and universal nature." Or, to put it in another way, people need to experience "that we are in God and God is in us" (244–45).

These deeply personal experiences are possible, says Kaplan, within the context of public worship. The seeming paradox of locating individual experience in a public setting grows out of a characteristic inherent in human nature. Kaplan labels this trait as the "gregarious instinct" and says that it "is of the very matrix of the spiritual life" (*Meaning of God*, 250). How does it work? Participation in public worship, when it goes well, dissolves the individual ego and allows one to experience "that power which, when moralized and ethicized, makes for cooperation" (250). So "religion does not end with experiencing the reality of God," rather "that is where it begins" (253). For Kaplan, religion in its fullness happens in community. Hence his strong interest in liturgy and group prayer: "No one can dispense with the experience of God that comes with public worship" (253). The individual, to live fully, must experience God within community; but without individual experience we don't have religion, only theology. Kaplan's life ethics, in short, requires that people work at keeping liturgy and public prayer alive and as relevant and aesthetically appealing as possible.

Another distinctive feature of Kaplan's life ethics stems from his conviction that "God is not known unless sought after" (*Meaning of God*, 30). This is one of the primary keys to salvation in Kaplan's ethics. For Kaplan, the truly religious person is a spiritual seeker. And where does one go seeking? One might expect Kaplan to send us to religious texts or to meditation. While these things are helpful they are, for him, only training grounds for the real search. The real search happens in the "midst of participation in human affairs and strivings" (30), and it is in the midst of this, in the realm of "ethical" experience, that we are truly seeking God. We are God-seekers, Kaplan says, when "we explore truth, goodness and beauty to their uttermost reaches" (30). Importantly, God-seeking is also prayer, which Kaplan defines as "the utterance of those thoughts that imply either the actual awareness of God, or the desire to attain such awareness" (33). Equally important to Kaplan's notion of prayer is the emphasis on thanksgiving, the kind of prayer that celebrates the divine goodness and creativity in-dwelling in the universe. This type of prayer sustains faith and optimism.

Living Ethics Through Holy Days

Having thus introduced Kaplan's theology of immanence and the kind of ethics that derives from it, I will attempt in what follows to further highlight this "new" approach to Jewish tradition as it relates to the celebration of Sacred Days. Creation, Revelation and Salvation are the three important themes on which I will focus. I choose these themes not only because they are of importance to Kaplan, but also because they are at the center of traditional Judaism. By examining his treatment of these themes in the context of *Meaning*'s reconception of the *luach*, we can glimpse what is different about Kaplan's approach to ethics.

Creation: The Sabbath. The Sabbath is the first of the traditional Jewish Holy Days. It is observed weekly, and may be said to stand for the key values of Judaism. The Sabbath traditionally celebrates the creation of the world by God, the Creator of all. In the pre-modern Jewish world, God the Creator is understood in transcendental terms, and the motif of transcendence is constantly repeated throughout the Sabbath liturgy. As I mention above, God the transcendental Creator is not part of Kaplan's immanentist paradigm. Here then, with the first of the traditional Sacred Days, Kaplan's deconstruction-reconstruction of Judaism may be said to begin.

His first step is to read the traditional sources on the Sabbath so that the day of rest comes to be seen as a symbol of the world's capacity to help people achieve this-worldly salvation: "the Sabbath implies an affirmation that the world is so constituted as to afford man the opportunity for salvation" (*Meaning of God*, 60). What is it about the world that makes such salvation possible? Kaplan's answer centers on the Hebrew phrase that refers to the Sabbath as *zeker lema'aseh bereshit*, "a reminder of the work of creation" (60). Traditionally this is related to the story of creation in the first chapter of Genesis. Kaplan, as pragmatist-immanentist, sees this story as a mythical account the Sabbath as a social institution. He likewise rejects the possibility and the need to gain information about the origin of the universe. For Kaplan, the modern Sabbath is "a means of accentuating the fact that we must reckon with creation and self renewal as a continuous process" (62). He reads the phrase *zeker lema'aseh bereshit* as "a reminder of the process of creativity" (62), rather than as a reminder of the once-and-for-all-time Creation of the universe by the transcendental God. Kaplan's Sabbath transforms transcendental Creation into the "conception of the creative urge as the element of Godhood in the world" (62).

This has ethical implications. In Kaplan's organismic life ethics, humans are seen as beings who naturally recreate themselves. Kaplan speaks about the inherent "yearning for spiritual self-regeneration" (*Meaning of God*, 62) that humans experience. He believes that this natural urge for self-renewal or self-recreation can be blunted unless protected and cultivated; it can, he says, "die down unless it is backed by the conviction that there is something which answers to it in the very character of life as a whole" (62). It is this conviction, then, that is renewed on every Sabbath, for according to Kaplan, "[t]he moral implication of the traditional teaching that God created the world is that creativity, or the continuous emergence of aspects of life not prepared for or determined by the past, constitutes the most divine phase of reality" (62). The last part of the statement needs highlighting because it refers to what might be called radical creativity, "the divine phase of reality" (62), as Kaplan puts it. He defines radical creativity as "the emergence of aspects of life not prepared for or determined by the past" (62). Radical creativity is the notion that creativity is not bound by cause and effect. Creativity is such that brand new results can be generated in the present that are not in any way related to the past.

The Sabbath, for Kaplan, should make people aware of the radical creativity operative within people and within nature overall. To effect this awareness requires the artistic and creative use of Sabbath liturgy and of community religious celebration, he suggests. Relevant here is Kaplan's idea that the individual needs community in order to be reminded, and thereby to be made aware of, the possibility of radical creativity. Awareness of radical creativity is so important that it needs to be brought to the center of the tradition on a weekly basis. Hence the Sabbath. This Holy Day is a sacred reminder of the human capacity for radical creativity.

Revelation: Shavuot. For traditional Judaism, revelation is threefold: God reveals laws; makes moral demands; enters into promises with His people. Traditional Judaism sees this threefold revelation as culminating on Mount Sinai, where, in a singular event, the transcendent God meets Moses and gives him the Torah, the moral law. The traditional notion is *Torah min hashamayim*, Torah given from above, from the transcendental realm known as heaven. The early summer festival of *Shavuot* celebrates the revelatory Sinai event.

For Kaplan, however, application of modern historiography and academic Biblical studies leads to the conclusion that the Sinai event is a myth. The traditional story has to be re-read and related to a new, modern, theory of revelation and of moral law. Revelation, says Kaplan, has to be tied to the intuition that there is an energy or power incessantly at work in the universe, and that this indwelling power, rather than a law delivered from above, is what motivates people to righteousness. Through extensive review of Biblical sources, especially Prophetic sources, Kaplan finds support for his thesis that revelation is ongoing and that morality is immanent, that it emanates from the revelatory force or power that is at work in the universe. The experience of God is the experience of this moral power. Hence, the word "God" gives symbolic expression to "the highest ideals for which men strive and at the same time, points to the objective fact that the world is so constituted as to make for the realization of those ideals" (*Meaning of God*, 306). These ideals are not simply humanist values. Kaplan argues strongly against atheistic humanism such as that espoused by Yirmiyahu Yovel, who speaks of people as value-creating beings but who does not believe that created values are inherent in the world. Kaplan challenges atheistic humanism just as much as he does traditional Judaism: both are missing the soterical God-idea: "God defined as the Power that endorses what we believe ought to be, and that guarantees that it will be" (324–25).

In keeping with his soterical approach, Kaplan defines right and wrong as cosmic categories, that is, categories which are held in common by all human social groups. Although the particulars may differ from one society to another, no society, he says, is without notions of the morally right and the morally wrong. Humans are the kinds of beings who are always seeking to understand right and wrong. The universality of this questioning is what, for Kaplan, points to a power beyond ourselves that impels us to seek righteousness. It "points to a power that makes for righteousness" (*Meaning of God*, 309). This aspect of God, God as immanent source of the search for righteousness, gives moral law the authority that a humanist ethics lacks. And "without such authority the moral law is without foundation" (309), an awareness that religious holidays are supposed to inculcate.

God is Not Known Unless Sought After. Religious observances are essential occasions of this search. The injunction to *Seek God!*, especially through observance of the Sacred Days, is another way in which Kaplan's ethics is distinguished from the atheistic humanisms of his day. But why *Shavuot*? Why are the symbols and myths of *Shavuot* necessary to Kaplan's ethics? His response would be that the observances of *Shavuot* provide people with the courage they need to deal with suffering and disappointment. *Shavuot* strengthens faith and inner resolve.

Let us return to the Sinai story. Traditional Judaism, when it retells the Sinai story, believes that God literally spoke on Sinai. In traditional tellings, revelation is a definitive event of *God speaking* to humans. But in Kaplan's paradigm, I have suggested, revelation is not centered on the pole of transcendence. Revelation is the result of human activity of God-seeking. Does it follow from this that in Kaplan's ethics, God no longer speaks or addresses us? At first glance the answer is, Kaplan's God does not speak. If we consider the issue more carefully, however, the answer is not a simple yes or no. Kaplan's is a process theology within which humans play a decisive role; humans are players in the ongoing process of revelation. Part of their role is to *give voice* to the energies and forces that Kaplan calls God. This voicing cannot happen without the search for God. As humans search, they articulate approximations of the reality they discover. As insights and realities change, so do the approximations that are, for Kaplan, revelations of the immanent voice of God. *Shavuot* and its symbols and story of Sinai are poetic reminders of the need to seek God and give voice to the Force called God.

Salvation: Rosh Hashannah, Yom Kippur, Sukkot. The terms "salvation" and "redemption" have Hebrew equivalents, *geulah* and *yeshuah*. Very often the Hebrew terms carry eschatological and apocalyptic overtones. These are in keeping with the idea of divine sovereignty that is at the heart of traditional Judaism's concept of salvation. The prophets and the Talmudic Rabbis looked forward to perfection of the world, as required by their sovereign God. It appears that sovereignty also became closely associated in Judaism with apocalypticism. Biblical books such as Daniel and Ezekiel depict the ultimate triumph of God's sovereignty in an end-event preceded by great cataclysmisms of various sorts: the rise of ruthless and oppressive leaders, large scale wars and nature catastrophes such as famine and pestilence (Ezekiel 38–39; Zechariah 14; Daniel 12:1). In Kaplan's case, however, "salvation" has a very this-worldly meaning; it implies self-fulfilment or self-realization. Ultimately, he seems to have replaced the term "salvation" with the word "soterics." Yet, most Kaplan commentators continue to use "salvation" in reference to his work. And of the three traditional categories, creation, revelation, salvation, the latter plays the largest part in *Meaning of God*. Salvation is the pivotal concept and it generates Kaplan's life ethics.

Kaplan, as a philosopher of finitude, predicts no final, cataclysmic human end and no natural upheavals (*Meaning of God*, 120). His version of modern Jewish religion cannot accept any such eschatological notions except as mythic expressions of hope. Yet, as a functionalist, he does not totally dismiss the value of apocalyptic mythology when it is viewed historically. Kaplan argues that traditional salvation mythology did provide hope and allow for meaningful survival. Jews, in the midst of vast social crises, "beheld the hand of God in those world-wide calamities" (142). Apocalyptic visions kept alive the hope and yearning for the arrival of the Kingdom of God, for divine salvation for Jewish people. Having said this, I have to add that Kaplan's treatment of sovereignty emphasizes hope, the ongoing and open-ended, rather than some final and fearful end.

The Sacred Days most closely related to sovereignty are *Rosh Hashannah* and *Yom Kippur*. These come in early Fall, as a ten day period during which it is believed that God literally judges the world. On these days, Jews are called to repent and to seek forgiveness so that God can render the most favorable judgement. The liturgy of these days emphasizes the Kingship of God and God's role as the sovereign Judge of all creation. As we would expect, Kaplan's immanentism leads him to interpret God's sovereignty not as a static state that will be achieve a once-and-for-all resolution for creation, but rather as a process-goal whose actualization is continuous and un-ending. The Kingdom of God, for Kaplan, is always and only *coming*.

Kaplan, it will be remembered, sees God as the creativity inherent in the universe. This divine energy not only creates new things but also *regenerates* that which already exists. It is the extended notion of creativity as regeneration that Kaplan finds expressed in the metaphor of the Kingdom of God. The coming of the Kingdom bespeaks renewal—and renewal of righteousness at that. Kaplan makes it clear that the Kingdom of God refers to this-worldly social, political and economic structures, and that regeneration is an entirely this-worldly enterprise. The Kingdom of God, as a metaphor, suggests "the regeneration of society by direct human agency, without reliance on an illusory hope of miraculous intervention" *(Meaning of God*, 109–110). Again, it must be remembered that, for Kaplan, God is the power that enables social regeneration to take place; but also that without human input, this renewing power could not effect social change. God, Kaplan concludes, "operates through individual humans" (110). It is clear, then, that for him, ethical religion requires that humans work together to better, to regenerate, the existing social order. Social responsibility is not separate from religion, and it does not operate independently of creation, revelation, and salvation.

The holy days of *Rosh Hashannah* and *Yom Kippur* emphasize the notion of *teshuvah*, repentance, return to God. In Kaplan's immanentist paradigm, such "returning" cannot be to a transcendent God, or even to the moral law of such a

God. And neither can the concept of sin be understood by Kaplan in transcendent, authoritarian terms. Both his notions of sin and of *teshuvah* have a "positive" ethical character that can best be got at through the word "responsibility." Sin, on a personal level, for example, has to do with not attending to caring and cultivating of one's inner self, one's soul. Our responsibility is to spiritual self-care, which takes place in three major steps: integration of the elements of self; continuous growth and development of self; cultivation of our own potentialities. These three steps are at the same time ethical principles conducive to a coherent, well-functioning life. Humans, in order to become morally whole, must respect all three of the principles. They are guidelines that give the measure of a person; also that, in Kaplan's process of *teshuvah*, enable a person, introspectively, to take stock of him/herself. The introspective exercise is what Kaplan sees as one of the major goals of both *Rosh Hashannah* and *Yom Kippur* (*Meaning of God*, 181–185).

Here, we return in a way to our starting point: that regeneration, as Kaplan understands it, is of the social dimension of human existence, something that requires the vigilance and sustained effort of responsible people. Such socially responsible selves need to undergo the process of *teshuvah*, which leads in turn to "the regeneration of human nature" (186). Both the individual and the community are energized by this process; both share in the creative and regenerative powers that are expressions of Godhood. Kaplan sees the recreation of the individual and the regeneration of society as two sides of the same process. Hence, he writes that "ethical religion is incompatible with an attitude of submission to social institutions that work injustice" (186). Humans work together with immanent divinity to drive the development of the Kingdom of God.

Such working together is especially imperative where economic justice is concerned. For Kaplan, economic justice is a cardinal religious and ethical value precisely because economics is "basic and determinative" of all other aspects of social life (*Meaning of God*, 209). At the basis of economic justice is that aspect of Godhood that makes for cooperation and without which there would be no mutual relations, no social life at all. Basic to economic justice, says Kaplan, is God, the power that makes cooperation possible. So important is this enabling power that Kaplan declares it to be a "literal fact" that only when God's power is manifest in our midst, can justice be appreciated and achieved (210).

Human living, then, is the work of God, the cosmic Artist, who exists in a unique kinship with humans.[4] Or, to put it in another way, human being, for Kaplan, is a dimension of the indwelling sacred Godhood. He argues that this sacredness of human being is the actual source of human rights, that "the recognition of the sacredness of personality carries with it the acknowledgment of rights of personality" (*Meaning of God*, 210). Kaplan goes on to consider ways in which human personality has developed over time, and he concludes that the very evolution of personality is "an expression of the immanence of God" (214). Since, in his view, "society is the matrix in which the very substance of personality is formed and nurtured," we are required to create a social order based on cooperation and equality (214–215). Kaplan does not believe that the principle of equality requires that all members have identical opportunities, but only "that all have an equal claim to the opportunity to pursue" life's opportunities within "the limits of their own varying capacities and in accordance with their own individual interests" (217). Godhood, he says, stands against those aspects of civilization that impede equality, so understood.

This is a point that Kaplan draws out of the Jewish Thanksgiving, *Sukkot*. His interpretation of *Sukkot*'s importance for the ethics of economic justice focuses on the festival's *sancta* or major symbols: the *Sukkah*, the booth and the ritual of thanksgiving; the waving of the *lulab* and *etrog*, the palm cluster and the citron fruit. In the traditional celebration of this Holy Day, Jews build a make-shift booth or shelter whose roof they cover with branches. During the seven-day festival of *Sukkot*, people eat, sleep and socialize in this shelter, called a *Sukkah*. The ancient custom has been explained in different ways. Kaplan sees the *Sukkah* ritual as related to an ancient sentiment which glorified the Wilderness period in Jewish history. In this ancient understanding, the *Sukkah* becomes a call to return to the mythological simplicity of desert life, a life not marred by the "artificialities and injustices of current civilization" (*Meaning of God*, 209). The biblical prophets, Kaplan suggests, created this mythology of desert purity and projected onto it the ideals of social and economic justice which they found lacking in their world. "Viewed in this light," he writes, "the *Sukkah* becomes the symbol of protest against the injustices and inequities of current civilization." The practice of "seating in the *Sukhah*" becomes an imaginative exercise in stepping outside the flow of ordinary life and entering the world of prophetic vision, a world established on the ideals of social and economic justice. This "time out" allows people, on return to the organized world, to demand the implementation of "standards of righteousness and justice" (208–209).

During *Sukkot*, tradition requires that thanksgiving prayers be offered. These prayers are accompanied by the shaking of the *lulab* and *etrog* in the six directions as a means of pointing to the natural forces that make food grow. As such, Kaplan suggests, the *lulab* ritual "emphasizes the need of making our economic life such that it will contribute to our joy in God" (*Meaning of God*, 29). The *sancta* here work in tandem: the *lulab* attests to the goodness of nature's bounty, while the *Sukhah* symbolizes the need to "so dispose of the income from

the resources of nature as to make . . . economic life conform to the social re-
lations that were obtained when Israel had not yet been contaminated by life in
Canaan" (210). The *Sukkot* ritual invokes the evil of an unjust society even as it
inspires the resolve to create a cooperative, economically just, social order (210).
For all these reasons, Kaplan says, *Sukkot* embodies the reality of God as the
Power That Makes For Cooperation.

Conclusion

I will return here to *Pesach*, Passover, as a final illustration of how Kaplan and his
associates reinterpreted or reconstructed the *luach*, the Sacred Calendar. As
discussed earlier, the Exodus story, the emancipation of the Jews from slavery, is
part of the Jewish master-myth. The story is filled with drama and with tales of
many miracles. One of the most famous of the miracles is the miracle of the ten
plagues visited on the land of Egypt. The last, the death of the first born among
the Egyptians, finally broke Pharaoh's resistance, and he then allowed the Hebrew
slaves to leave the bondage of Egypt. The Exodus story forms the core of the
Passover festival meal, which is widely observed by Jews throughout the world.
It is called a *Seder*, because it has a specific format or order for telling the story
of freedom through use of symbols, prayer, music and even dance. The major
symbolic items are foodstuffs, most of which are eaten in a ceremonial fashion.

Rabbi Ira Eisenstein, a first generation disciple of Kaplan's, has written a
popular version of *The Meaning of God in Modern Jewish Religion* entitled *What
We Mean By Religion*. He points out, as does Kaplan, that Passover was originally
a widespread Spring harvest festival which the aboriginal peoples of ancient
Canaan, ancient Palestine, celebrated. When the Hebrews came to Canaan, they
too adopted this Springtime harvest festival. Eventually, the Hebrews added to
this nature-oriented festival the remembrance of their liberation from Egypt,
which took place in the Spring. It "became a kind of double celebration; but
throughout Jewish history our ancestors always thought of Passover as, first and
foremost, the Festival of Freedom" (Eisenstein, *What We Mean By Religion*,
124–25). But how does Eisenstein, following Kaplan, understand Passover and its
rituals? Of course, he rejects the supernatural and miraculous elements,
understanding "freedom" as a manifestation of the cosmic Force that makes for
salvation: "*Pesach* teaches us . . . that there is a Power in us that seeks freedom,
and a Power in the world that helps us remember that freedom is precious."
Moreover, "*Pesach* teaches us . . . that God, the Power in the world that makes us
continually seek freedom, will not let us rest until the goal has been reached"
(135). Traditionally, Passover focused on the emancipation of the Jews. But

Kaplan and Eisenstein find in Passover a double message: freedom for Jews to live out their cultural and religious lives, and the liberation of all peoples. On the latter point, Eisenstein, like Kaplan, adds a significant caveat: "the freedom of the Jewish people today cannot be achieved unless all the persecuted peoples of the world are also set free" (126). After all, God, as the Power that makes for Freedom, flows through the entire universe.

In 1941, Kaplan along with Eisenstein and Eugene Kohn published a revised rendition of the Passover Seder ritual entitled *The New Haggadah*. It attempts to preserve the traditional framework but also to fill it with the living, compelling content of present day idealism and aspiration. The old and new materials are aimed at the young American Jew, in whom, it is hoped, a reconstructed tradition will stir the devotion to freedom that his/her Jewish ancestors gained from the traditional celebration. While the traditional Biblical story is told, and while all the traditional symbols are present, *The New Haggadah* all but eliminates supernatural and miraculous elements.

The story of the plague, for instance, is not used. Another example has to do with the green herb. Usually, the Seder table has on it parsley or lettuce or some other green herb which is dipped in salt water. Traditional interpretations of the dipping ceremony ignore the symbolism of herb and explain that the salt water represents the tears of the Hebrew slaves. *The New Haggadah* reverses this emphasis by relating the green herb to the coming of Spring: "these greens symbolize the coming of Spring and suggest the perpetual renewal of life, and hence, the ever-sustaining hope of human redemption" (*The New Haggadah*, xi). In keeping with their philosophical naturalism, the editors reintroduce nature to the consciousness of their audience. They also present the theme of universal human redemption. Yet another example concerns the wine: four times during the *Pesach* Seder meal, the wine cup is filled. This traditionally related to the four promises given by God to the Hebrew slaves. In *The New Haggadah*, however, the filling of the cups is prefaced by an invocation that remembers the ancient story but that also calls our attention to the suffering of all those alive today. The wine-filling ritual ends with a universalistic prayer: "let us pray that the time be not distant when all the world will be liberated from cruelty, tyranny, oppression and war" (3).

This rewriting of the Passover Seder service illustrates the manner in which Kaplan and his followers attempt to give poetic and artistic expression to the philosophy of immanence, and how the resulting rituals differ in intent and content from traditional or orthodox approaches to Sacred Days. Kaplan's version of Jewish religion can be summarized as follows:

• *God/Godhood* is the Force at work in the universe. This Force supports the ethical, creative and artistic aspects of human life.

• *Torah* is the record of the Jewish people's search for God and of their visions of a world fashioned according to their image of God.

• *Israel* refers to the Jews as a "people" or a "civilization" with a distinctive cultural and religious history. These people have undergone considerable change and have changed their God-idea. For all their distinctiveness, Jews are not "chosen," but are one people among many others.

Postscript

Kaplan began his Seminary classes with a prayer, sometimes traditional, sometimes creative. He was a man of prayer as he understood prayer. His many journals, the ones that I noticed all around his chair when I visited him in Jerusalem, are filled with his prayers.

In doing the research for this essay, I visited the Kaplan Archive in Philadelphia, Pennsylvania. I found there the following prayer that Kaplan wrote at the time of the birth of a grandchild. Here, too, he addresses God as he understands God. I am quoting the prayer exactly as I saw it:

> This morning at 10:38 Hadassah gave birth to a son. May God grant Judith as easy a parturition. She expects her baby sometime in April.
> God (the sum of those processes that make life worthwhile and significant) has been, to use the conventional parlance, mighty good to me and my family. Would to God that all human beings had occasion to be as happy and grateful as I am (December 3, 1935).

Notes

1. In recent scientific and theological writing much is made of the Anthropic Principle, the notion that the structure of the universe is such that it supports human existence and human life (Gould, 397; McFague, 75). In 1937, when Kaplan published *Meaning*, this term was unknown. Yet, Kaplan seems to have articulated a version of the Anthropic Principle: "reality is so constituted as to endorse and guarantee the realization in man of that which is of greatest value to him." Kaplan sees his "Anthropic Principle" as an article of faith, that is, a belief which is "not susceptible of proof." Kaplan says that believing this means "we have faith in God." This, writes Kaplan, is the only bit of metaphysical speculation we as people need (*Meaning of God*, 29).

2. While Kaplan, as an immanentist, understands religion in general and Judaism in particular, as the product of naturalistic forces and historical evolution, he is quick to point out that although the idea of God has changed over time, much of the vocabulary of the divine has remained the same. Why is this so? The retention of established religious terminology (and ritual), derives from the basic human need of feeling continuity, he suggests. Further, there is a distinct advantage in reinterpreting traditional concepts because, Kaplan says, "they carry with them the accumulated momentum and emotional drive of man's previous efforts to attain greater spiritual power (*Judaism as a Civilization*, 386). In *Greater Judaism in the Making*, Kaplan claims that the transcendentalized Judaism points to some of the most important religious and spiritual realities, but that the outmoded transcendentalist thought system uses the wrong referents for these experiences; they spelled "the name of God with the wrong idea blocks."

3. In my imagination I can hear immanentist philosopher Yovel bristling and calling Kaplan either a "dogmatic immanentist," or worse, a "soft transcendentalist." All of which may be true. But for our purposes it seems more helpful to say that Kaplan's Anthropic Principle is what philosopher Ben-Ami Scharfstein calls an "experiential axiom." These are fundamental assumptions which many different types of philosophers and scientists come to based on powerful experiences which are then translated into foundational axioms. I come to this conclusion largely based on the observations found in J. J. Cohen's recent book on Kaplan and Abraham Yitzchah Kok, *Morim Lezaman Nevuchim* (1993).

4. Kaplan brought to his revisioning of Jewish religion the claim that traditional Judaism placed little or no positive value on art and the artist. In *Meaning*, he advocates raising the profile of the art and the artist in Jewish life. In discussing the manner in which the cosmic creative process has showily formed the world of culture, art, science, and religion, Kaplan also speaks of God as an artist, as a sculptor, to be exact: "The sculptor with his chisel in hand stands before a block of marble and begins to hew. Presently there emerges the outline of a human form. After a while we behold distinct features of a face, in which we recognize character." God, "the great world Artist," continues this hewing "until there gradually emerge human souls, each stamped with an individuality of its own" (*Meaning of God*, 281–82). If God is the "great world Artist" who deliberately works at fashioning the human being, then what better metaphor for the goal which Kaplan's ethics set for humans, than to master the "art of living." Kaplan tells us that "the distinctive achievement of the Jewish spirit" is the insight it has discovered into converting "living into an art" Jewish ethics is "the art of living" (188).

Works Cited

Eisenstein, Ira. 1946. *What We Mean By Religion.* New York: Behrman House Inc.

Cohen, J. J. 1993. *Morim Lezaman Nevuchim.* Tel-Aviv: Akod Press.

Goldsmith, Emanuel, S. and Mel Schult, eds. 1985. *Dynamic Judaism: The Essential Writings of Mordecai M. Kaplan.* New York: Fordham University Press/Reconstructionist Press.

Goldsmith, Emanuel, S. M. Schult, and R. Seltzer, eds. 1990. *The American Judaism of Mordecai Kaplan.* New York: New York University Press.

Gould, Steven. 1981. *The Flamingo's Smile.* New York: W. W. Norton.

Kaplan, Mordecai. 1996. *Not So Random Thoughts.* New York: Reconstructionist Press.

————. 1960. *Greater Judaism in the Making.* New York: Reconstructionist Press.

————. 1958. *Judaism Without Supernaturalism.* New York: Reconstructionist Press.

————. 1948. *The Future of the American Jew.* New York: MacMillan.

————. 1937. *The Meaning of God in Modern Jewish Religion.* New York: Reconstructionist Press.

————. 1934. *Judaism as a Civilization.* New York: MacMillan.

Kaplan, Mordecai, M., Ira Eisenstein and Eugene Kohn. 1941. *The New Haggadah.* New York: Behrman House Inc.

McFague, Sallie. 1993. *The Body of God.* Minneapolis: Fortress Press.

Scharfstein, Ben-Ami. 1980. *Philosophers and Their Lives.* New York: Oxford.

Yovel, Yirmiyahu. 1989. *Spinoza and Other Heretics.* Princeton: Princeton University Press.

Chapter 7

Bernard J. F. Lonergan: Existential Ethics

David G. Creamer

The Issue of Contraception

Within the Christian tradition, contraception has been and still is a contentious issue, especially within the Roman Catholic church. Our approach will be to set forth the traditional position on this issue and then, drawing on the existential ethics of Bernard Lonergan, consider how modern science, historical criticism, and contemporary conceptions of personhood have each elaborated upon the traditional view, providing us with a plurality of competing opinions about an issue that once seemed so clear and certain. Then, from our consideration of the debate *out there*, we will again use Lonergan to move *inwards* to consider how an existential subject might come to a personal decision on an ethical issue such as contraception. So as not to complicate the example unnecessarily, we will limit our consideration of contraception to *artificial* means of birth control and for the most part focus on the continuing debate and discussion with Roman Catholicism where the issue is still very much alive.[1]

The traditional Christian attitude towards the use of artificial means of birth control is quite clear: artificial contraception is always wrong because it is opposed to natural law (i.e., God's law). Even after the Protestant Reformation this traditional attitude endured, for in post-Reformation Christianity, birth control, unlike some other questions, did not become a Catholic-Protestant issue. All mainline Christian churches took a stand against contraception. Contraception became a contentious issue only on August 14, 1930 when the Lambeth Conference of Anglican Bishops overturned their earlier consistent teaching on the immorality of contraception and reluctantly gave a qualified acceptance of marital contraception. In the United States, this decision was followed up by a 1931

Federal Council of Churches endorsement of "the careful and restrained use of contraceptives by married people."

The reaction of the Roman Catholic church to these developments was swift and pointed. Pope Pius XI's encyclical, *Casti Connubii*, published on December 31, 1930, made specific reference to the Lambeth resolution:

> Since, therefore, openly departing from the uninterrupted Christian tradition some recently have judged it possible solemnly to declare another doctrine regarding this question, the Catholic Church . . . proclaims anew: any use whatsoever of matrimony exercised in such a way that the act is deliberately frustrated in its natural power to generate life is an offense against the law of God and of nature, and those who indulge in such are branded with the guilt of a grave sin. [# 56]

The encyclical states the traditional foundation of the teaching in natural law as follows:

> no reason, however grave, may be put forward by which anything intrinsically against nature may be conformable to nature and morally good. Since, therefore, the conjugal act is destined primarily by nature for the begetting of children, those who in exercising it deliberately frustrate its natural power and purpose sin against nature and commit a deed which is shameful and intrinsically vicious. [# 54]
>
> Even by the light of reason alone and particularly if the ancient records of history are investigated, if the unwavering popular conscience is interrogated and the manners and instructions of all races examined, it is sufficiently obvious that there is a certain sacredness and religious character attaching even to the purely natural union of man and woman, "not something added by chance but innate, not imposed by men but involved in the nature of things." [# 80]

Notwithstanding *Casti Connubii* and subsequent Vatican pronouncements, with the advent of the birth control pill in the 1960's, artificial contraception was almost universally practiced by most family planners (including many Roman Catholics).

Nevertheless, in 1968, Pope Paul VI issued his controversial encyclical *Humanae Vitae* which reaffirmed the traditional Catholic prohibition of the use of artificial means of birth control for all married couples in all circumstances: "the Church, calling men back to the observance of the norms of natural law, as interpreted by the constant doctrine, teaches that each and every marriage act (*quilibet matrimonii usus*) must remain open to the transmission of life" [# 11]. The encyclical goes on: "excluded is every action which, either in anticipation of the conjugal act, or in its accomplishment, or in the development of its natural consequences, proposes, whether as an end or as a means, to render procreation impossible" [# 14].

Pope Paul VI was well aware that his teaching would "not be easily received by all" but his position was that he had a "grave responsibility" to speak what he believed to be the truth, not what was popular. A great debate raged within the Catholic church and today most Roman Catholics have chosen, often after agonizing soul-searching, to demur from the official teaching. American priest/sociologist, Andrew Greeley, reports that after its publication, only 15% of lay Catholics and priests in the United States accepted *Humanae Vitae*. According to the American 1988 Survey of Family Growth, only 3% of married Catholic couples doing anything at all about family planning were using any form of Natural Family Planning. In 32% of those studied, one or other of the partners was sterilized, 34% were using the Pill, and 25% were using condoms or inter-uterine devices.[2]

How can these ethical decisions be interpreted? This paper turns to Bernard Lonergan for help in answering this question.

Who is Bernard Lonergan?

Bernard Lonergan (1904–1984) is a Canadian Jesuit philosopher and theologian who devoted most of his life to the elaboration of an integrated and generalized method of inquiry which he saw as able to overcome Catholic focus on the syllogistic logic of medieval Scholasticism as well as modern divisions and fragmentation in knowledge. As Lonergan studied and taught in Rome and Canada, he came to a deepening awareness that the Christian philosophical and theological tradition, in which he had been formed, needed more openness to modern ways of looking at things. Nowhere was this shift more evident than in the area of ethics where the natural law tradition, with its affirmation of absolute, universal, and unchanging norms for behavior was assailed by scientific probability, a growing consciousness of personal freedom, and a new under-standing of the historical process. And so, as Bernard Lonergan finished his doctoral studies at the Gregorian University in Rome, he committed himself to nothing less than the total reconstruction of both philosophy and theology. *Insight: A Study of Human Understanding* (1957) and *Method in Theology* (1972) are the major fruits of that effort.

Without denigrating the genuine achievements of the past, Lonergan sought to elaborate the intellectual justification for a decisive shift in focus, away from static and absolute truths to the existential *experience* of the believer who affirms truth. For too long, he argued, Christian thinkers subordinated the realities of human life to seven century old Scholastic formulations that had become *the* formulations. We subordinated *living* life to *knowing* truth, subordinated human experience to the demands of static propositions.

It was clear to Bernard Lonergan that an acceptance of the "new learning" in science, history, and the human sciences demands the rethinking of everything, yet in a manner that *preserves a continuity* with the genuine achievements of the tradition (let us not throw out the baby with the bath water) and in a manner that enables us to judge precisely what is genuinely going forward from those achievements. For Lonergan, a key component in this shift from the classical to modern world view is the "recovery" of the human subject who experiences, understands, judges, decides, and loves. Lonergan's approach to ethics, then, is to discover in human existence the foundation for ethical affirmation.

Because Bernard Lonergan's theory of ethics is an extension of his theory of knowledge (ethics is only possible if knowledge of truth is possible) we need to begin with knowing.

Human Knowing

Lonergan's analysis is of human intentional acts of experiencing, imagining, remembering, desiring, wondering, inquiring, understanding, conceiving, reflecting, evaluating, judging, deliberating, deciding, acting, and loving. More simply, Lonergan sought to clarify and unfold a methodological answer to the question 'What does it mean to know?'

Our initial focus, then, will be Lonergan's answers to the question 'What am I doing when I am knowing?' Then, we will focus on ethical questions—'How do I know what is really worthwhile?' 'How am I to decide what to make of myself?' The answers to these questions are at the heart of Lonergan's existential ethics.

What am I doing when I am knowing?

Bernard Lonergan's investigation into the dynamics of human cognition led him to propose that all conscious and intentional operations of knowing occur by means of a dynamic interlocking pattern of experiencing, understanding, judging, and deciding.

Using a spacial metaphor, Lonergan speaks of four *levels* through which the dynamic of conscious intentionality unfolds: the *empirical* level of conscious attention to the external data, characterized by the operations of our senses (seeing, hearing, touching, smelling, tasting) and including as well the internal data provided by consciousness (perceiving, imagining, anticipating, feeling, remembering); the *intellectual* level of consciousness, characterized by inquiry, insight (the act of understanding) and conceptualizing;[3] the *rational* level of consciousness, characterized by all operations of reflecting and weighing the evidence which are involved in verifying our understanding and judging the truth of what is; and the *responsible* level of consciousness characterized by deliberating, evaluating, and deciding about what good action ought to be done. This process brings us to a knowledge of reality, knowledge of what *is*.

In ordinary daily life when we ask someone 'How do you know?' and they respond with a definitive 'Because I saw it!' the issue is normally settled. We often behave as if the real world is what we can plainly "see" if we just take a good look (naive realism) or, in a more sophisticated manner, as if the real is what we *know* through sense experience (empiricism). Lonergan does not claim that the empirical point of view is wrong, only that it is incomplete; it takes just one of the components of knowing (experiencing) and treats it as if it were the whole of knowing. Knowing, for Lonergan, is the object of judgments and decisions made in light of our understanding of given data of experience. Inquiry, insight, formulation, reflection, judgment, truthfulness, goodness, trust, fidelity, caring, and love cannot be grasped by means of the senses and are therefore pejoratively labeled "subjective" (unreliable) by empiricists, yet these activities are at the very *heart* of the knowing process.

A concrete illustration of cognitional theory may serve to consolidate our appropriation of the unfolding of what Lonergan refers to as the "generalized empirical method." Consider how television star Peter Falk, as Lieutenant Columbo, solves a murder case. What is unusual about a *Columbo* mystery is that at the outset we see the murder being planned and executed; we know who did it, as well as when, where, and how. Over the time remaining, we see Lieutenant Columbo's painstaking efforts to collect and assess evidence. His detective work moves from cigar puffing and head scratching at the complexity of the clues through a logical series of questions for intelligence: What happened? Why is this here? How does this fit? Where did that come from? Who could have done that? Columbo records *data* in his little black book, checks and double-checks, struggling to fathom how seemingly random pieces of evidence fit together. He goes off on tangents but endless questions raise suspicions and solve small puzzles until the parts form a whole, the penny drops, and a flash of *insight* gives him an idea. As he continues to scratch his head, search for matches in his shabby coat, and drive around in his old car, he surfaces questions for reflection (Is that really so? Am I certain?) and forms and tests hypotheses. Methodically, Columbo builds a case until he arrives at a possible, then probable, and finally certain *judgment* as to the true identity of the guilty party. In the final scene, he makes the arrest. Since we viewers know the identity of the guilty party from the very beginning of the show, why do we bother to watch *Columbo*? In my view, it is because of our fascination with the dynamics of human knowing, with the relentlessness of the process of understanding the evidence and arriving at the precise judgment that fits all of the facts beyond any doubt. *Columbo*, Lonergan would say, gives us an insight into insight.

From what we have seen to this point, I think it is clear that human knowing is not a single activity but a dynamic *structure* or *set* of different but complementary activities. Each step in the generalized empirical method builds on the preceding one: without the data of experience there is no possibility of inquiry and understanding; without a proper grasp of intelligibility (relationships and meanings), correct judgment is impossible; without having made a judgment as to what is so, no proper decision as to what to do can be taken. According to Lonergan, as we achieve the goal of a particular level we go on, *spontaneously*, to the next. We are *impelled* to move from one level of consciousness to the next by wonder, by our intellectual curiosity, by means of that inborn human need to find answers to questions—all of which Lonergan calls our "detached, disinterested, unrestricted desire to know" (Lonergan, *Insight*, 659).[4]

What I reach as a result of conscious intentionality is a highly *probable* judgment; highly probable in that it is revisable in the light of further evidence. What I can do is make a *reasonable* affirmation as to what is the truth. So, even though what I achieve as a result of the process of experiencing, understanding, judging and deciding is not *absolute* certainty, neither am I left with the polar opposite extreme of mere opinion. What I reach **is** knowledge of *what is*. It **is** *truth*. I like to characterize what is known by this transcendental process as being *relatively* absolute!

In addition, truth, for Lonergan, is necessarily *my* truth; truth which *I* arrive at by means of the pattern of human consciousness expanding through empirical, intellectual, rational, and responsible levels. Truth is not something *apart* from me, carved into granite or preserved in an illuminated manuscript, passed down and accepted uncritically by subsequent generations, because, unless I have made it my own, it represents the work of another person's mind and comes to me secondhand. *I* do not yet know it as truth until the stone or manuscript become data I judge with sufficient evidence to be true in light of my own understanding and critical reflection.[5]

Despite the emphasis above on the words *my* and *I*, I trust that you can see why Bernard Lonergan is not open to the charge of relativism. The choice for

Lonergan is not between the *traditional* stance supporting eternal, unchanging, absolute truths and what many people take to be the *modern* view that truth is relative and so everything is just a matter of opinion. There is, he argues, a third alternative (critical realism); what is absolute or normative in knowing is *not* so much the *object* I am trying to know but the *process I follow* in coming to know. It is this *pattern* of my conscious and intentional operations which forms the "rock" on which I can build truth.

The dynamic of the generalized empirical method grounds what Lonergan calls the "transcendental precepts" which guide the gradual expansion of human consciousness: *Be attentive, Be intelligent, Be reasonable, Be responsible.* There is, he suggests, an imperative quality to the dynamics of human consciousness.

Note that the spontaneous drive operating at each level of consciousness is in the form of a *precept* or imperative and not *necessity.* Although we are called to be attentive to data, to probe intelligently, to reflect reasonably, and to decide responsibly, we need not respond to the call; we can choose to be inattentive, obtuse, unreasonable, and irresponsible. Human freedom lies in that capacity for choice.[6] Who among us cannot recall instances when we have known the right thing to do but have not done it! We *can* and at times *do* impede or derail the deepest desires of our minds and hearts.

These four interlocking levels constitute human consciousness and the *pattern* of the operations involved is *normative.*[7] This methodological "rock" is the foundation upon which a responsible ethics can be constructed.

As we follow the steps of the generalized empirical method, as we move from one level of human consciousness to another, the *quality* of our consciousness is enlarged. According to Lonergan, as we have seen, the data of philosophy (human consciousness) and the methodology used in doing it (intentionality analysis) are coincidental. As questions move us from level to level "it is a fuller self of which we are aware and the awareness itself is different" (Lonergan, *Method,* 9). We are conscious, not only that our cognitive operations and choices are different, but that *we* are different. In other words, more of ourselves, more of what it is to be human, is at risk as we go from experiencing to understanding to judging to deciding. As a professor correcting examination papers, for example, I find it quite easy to admit that through oversight I missed a student's answer or added up grades incorrectly. As students come to my office to discuss their work, it is a little more difficult to acknowledge that I have misunderstood them, and to concede that I misjudged their motives would necessitate an admission of some personal failure. Finally, to say that I made a mistake and followed a wrong course of action in my dealings with a student is tantamount to confessing to some serious flaw in my very character.

What is significant, for Lonergan, about the movement through the levels of consciousness, then, is not just the growing complexity of the operations involved but the change in ourselves as we move from receptivity, to inquiry, to verification, to ethical decision making:

> [As human beings] we are so endowed that we not only ask questions leading to self-transcendence, not only can recognize correct answers constitutive of intentional self-transcendence, but also respond with the stirring of our very being when we glimpse the possibility . . . of oneself as a moral being, the realization that one not only chooses between courses of action but also thereby makes oneself an authentic human being or an unauthentic one. (Lonergan, *Method*, 38)

By this point in our consideration of Lonergan's thought, he may look to you like an ivory-tower philosopher, offering incomprehensible answers to insoluble problems (to borrow a definition I heard somewhere). He was certainly aware that "in the minds of some" he dwelt in a "cocoon of abstractions" (Liddy, *Transforming Light*, 209). In my opinion, Lonergan *isn't* an abstract, ivory-tower thinker and, as this summary of his thought unfolds, *you* ought to be able to see the practicality of his approach.

Two Ways of Human Development

So far we have principally focused on the levels of consciousness as moving *upward* from experience to understanding to judgment to decision. But the fact is that we don't generally live our lives in this logical order. While affirming the creative process, Lonergan reminds us that human development is more "fundamentally" and more "importantly" a healing process from above downwards. It became progressively apparent to Bernard Lonergan that the single structure of human consciousness could be traversed in two complementary ways, inverse but complementary components of a *single structure* of human consciousness. What we must keep before us, then, as we reflect on human knowing is that it is not a question of either/or but of both/and—we learn *both* by means of the distinct but interdependent path from below upwards (way of achievement) *and* by means of the distinct but interdependent path from above downwards (way of tradition).

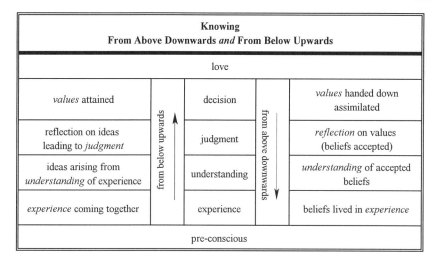

Knowing From Above Downwards *and* From Below Upwards				
love				
values attained		decision		*values* handed down assimilated
reflection on ideas leading to *judgment*		judgment		*reflection* on values (beliefs accepted)
ideas arising from *understanding* of experience		understanding		*understanding* of accepted beliefs
experience coming together		experience		beliefs lived in *experience*
pre-conscious				

There are serious limitations inherent in focusing on either way of knowing to the neglect of the other. If knowing was *only* conceived classically as preserving and passing on the wisdom of the past (from above downwards), there would be no such thing as progress. Carried to its extreme we would still be starting fire with flint. Yet, if knowing was *only* conceived empirically (dynamically, from below upwards) there would be constant change and development but there would be no sense of accumulating patrimony or wisdom. In its extreme there would be *nothing* classical; no classical music or art, no classic books or cars. As Lonergan puts it, "just as the creative process [from below upwards], when unaccompanied by healing, is distorted and corrupted by bias, so too the healing process [from above downwards], when unaccompanied by creating, is a soul without a body" (Lonergan, *Third Collection*, 107).

To turn for a moment to our contraception example, a Catholic is first expected to embrace the Christian message as found in Scripture, the Creed, the sacraments, and church teachings (way of tradition). Any talk of disagreement with the teaching on artificial birth control in *Humanae Vitae* (way of achievement) takes place in the context of fidelity to and respect for the church and its teaching office.

A recognition of the interdependence and balance between the two ways, therefore, is required for authenticity. We receive the traditions and wisdom of our ancestors which we adapt to the needs of our times and places; we live by it, we critique it, we modify it, we add to it, and we pass that enhanced knowledge on to the next generation.

Lonergan's Existential Ethics

*How am I to decide what is worthwhile to do? How am I to decide what to
make of myself?*

> by deliberate and responsible freedom we move beyond merely
> self-regarding norms and make ourselves moral beings.
> (Lonergan, *Third Collection*, 29)

Lonergan argues that as human beings we are more than mere *knowing*
subjects (mind), we are *agent*-subjects imbued with a built-in spontaneous drive
to seek congruence between what we know and what we do. So while knowledge
of the truth is *necessary* in ethical decision making, it is not *sufficient*: knowing
needs to be "subsumed under higher operations that integrate knowing with
feeling and consist of deliberating, evaluating, deciding, acting" (Lonergan,
Second Collection, 204).

On this fourth level of consciousness, that of conscience, we come face to
face with the basic ethical question: 'Why be moral at all?' 'Is doing the truth
worthwhile?' Lonergan would say that an affirmative answer to this question
presupposes "moral conversion"; i.e., presupposes that I desire to put the interests
of others ahead of my own, group satisfaction before personal satisfaction.
'What's in it for me?' gives way to 'What is really worthwhile?'

How do we arrive at this ethical decision-making level of human
consciousness? Just as questions calling for understanding move us from the
empirical to the intellectual level of consciousness, and questions for reflection
move us from the intellectual level to the level of judgment, so questions about
what would be truly good and worthwhile move us from the rational level to the
existential level, from consciousness to conscience. For Lonergan, the "nagging
conscience" keeps the basic ethical question before us and the "good conscience"
is the peace of mind that comes from knowing that we have chosen to do something truly worthwhile (Lonergan, *Third Collection*, 174).

There is in us "an internal compass," a fundamental or innate drive, targeted
to what is true and worthwhile, and we know when we have arrived there. Because
more than mind is involved in our "detached, disinterested, unrestricted desire to
know," we are drawn beyond cognition to a higher level of human consciousness
where affectivity (heart) joins with knowledge (head) in responsible decision-
making about the values by which we will live. To quote Blaise Pascal, as
Lonergan often does, "the heart has its reasons of which reason knows nothing"
(Pascal, *Pensées*, 154). "Without feelings this experience, understanding,

judgment," Lonergan asserts, "is paper-thin. The whole mass and momentum of living is in feeling" (Lonergan, *A Second Collection*, 221).

Affectivity, in fact, is at the center of the fourth level of human intending. It is critical to authenticity at this level; it is in feelings that possible values are *first* apprehended and it is largely in negotiating our feelings that ethical decision-making takes place. The addition of the affective dynamics of *heart* to the cognitional dynamics of *mind* leads to a corresponding shift in decision-making from doing what is reasonable to acting responsibly. We have seen that knowledge of what *is* flows from a pure detached, disinterested desire to know. As I make decisions about what I value, I am neither detached nor disinterested!

The dynamics of human consciousness, then, move us beyond *cognitional* questions of truth to *affective* questions of value, we desire to know because we want to act, and act responsibly. We pay attention to experience and consciousness, inquire intelligently into the meaning of our experience, and exercise critical judgment, because we want to make responsible decisions, thereby to become *moral*—"to become moral practically, for our decisions affect things; to become moral interpersonally, for our decisions affect other persons; to become moral existentially, for by our decisions we constitute what we are to be" (Lonergan, *Third Collection*, 29). The endpoint of the knowing process is ethical, *not* cognitional. We need to *know* the truth of a matter in order that we may *act* with justice and compassion.

Object-Pole in Ethical Decision-Making

In Lonergan's method, we must focus our attention in both knowing and doing on two centers; a subject-pole and an object-pole. The subject-pole is the conscious human person experiencing, understanding, and evaluating the data pertaining to a given ethical issue. The object-pole includes the total complex of data which the subject evaluates in coming to a decision. For Lonergan, the object-pole, in our contraception example, contains the data of Scripture and tradition, official church teaching, as well as the scholarship of contemporary theologians, but it also contains data from history, biology, sociology, theology, psychology, and so on. Through the use of the transcendental method the human subject seeks to understand and evaluate official church teaching in light of this complex of additional data to arrive at a personal decision as to the correct course of action to follow. We will consider a few examples of factual data which pertain to the issue of contraception in order to illustrate what Lonergan understands to be the content of the object-pole in ethical decision-making.

First, modern biological science has enlarged our understandings of human sexuality. Lonergan's letter on contraception and the natural law[8] summarizes this new scientific data very well:

> traditional Catholic doctrine on the sexual act followed rigorously from the position adopted by Aristotle in his *De generatione animalium*. That position was that the seed of the male was an instrumental cause that changed the matter supplied by the female into a sentient being. As was argued from the instance of wind-eggs, the female by herself got no further than a nutritive principle. The efficient causality of the male was needed to produce the sensitive principle or soul. On that basis it was clear that every act of insemination was of itself procreative and that any positive interference was an act of obstructing the seed in its exercise of its efficient causality.
>
> Two factors, however, have combined to bring about a notable change in the views of Catholic theologians on this matter. The first, of course, is the fact that the Aristotelian position is erroneous. Insemination and conception are known now to be quite distinct. The act of inseminating is not an act of procreating in the sense that of itself, per se, it leads to conception. The relation of insemination to conception is just statistical and, far more frequently than not, insemination does not lead to conception.
>
> So there arises the question whether this statistical relationship of insemination to conception is sacrosanct and inviolable. Is it such that no matter what the circumstances, the motives, the needs, any deliberate modification of the statistical relationship must always be prohibited? If one answers affirmatively, he is condemning the rhythm method. If negatively, he permits contraceptives in some cases. Like the diaphragm and the pill, the menstrual chart and the thermometer directly intend to modify the statistical relationship nature places between insemination and conception.

Second, historical criticism sheds light on the development of the traditional doctrine prohibiting artificial contraception and a weighing of this evidence may significantly affect one's personal decision about the matter. To illustrate the nature of this data relating to contraception, we will consider two examples from history, one ancient and one recent.

We now know that the development of the Christian natural law tradition in moral theology owes more to Greek philosophy and Roman law than to Jesus and biblical sources. Stoicism, popular among the upper classes at the time of Jesus, emphasized living life in conformity with the law given in nature. By the third century CE, Roman jurists distinguished between three types of law: *jus civile* which regulated the life of citizens within the state, *jus gentium* which regulated affairs between legally autonomous states, and *jus naturale* which was a generic law common to humans and animals. The influences of Stoicism and

Roman law gave Christian natural law ethics a *physicalist* cast; i.e., the moral act was identified with the physical act which corresponded to natural animal processes. What is most significant for our purposes is that the traditional teaching about the immorality of contraception is centered on the *sexual act*, on humans as more *like* than different from animals.

In 1963, because of ambiguities and uncertainties in the church about artificial birth control, Pope John XXIII established a six member Pontifical Birth Control Commission. Pope Paul VI later expanded that commission to sixty-seven people (a rather conservative collection of churchmen, scientists, doctors, theologians, and three married couples) and set them the task of studying the whole question and making *expert* recommendations. In 1966, the papal Birth Control Commission recommended *against* publishing a reaffirmation of *Casti Connubii*, as did the Pope's personal theologians, but after a delay of two years, Paul VI published *Humanae Vitae* which restated the traditional Catholic condemnation of artificial means of birth control.

A third type of data that impinges on a modern person trying to make an ethical decision about using artificial birth control has to do with our understanding of what it is to be a person. Traditionally the church taught that the primary purpose of marriage was procreation; love was a secondary and rather remote purpose of matrimony. The Second Vatican Council's *Pastoral Constitution on the Church in the Modern World* (*Gaudium et Spes*) offered a corrective to this one sided understanding of marriage in its affirmation of two equally important ends in marriage, the mutual love of the partners *and* the procreation and raising of children. This teaching is restated in the recent *Catechism of the Catholic Church*: "The matrimonial covenant, by which a man and a woman establish between themselves a partnership of the whole of life, is by its nature ordered toward the good of the spouses and the procreation and education of offspring . . ." (# 1601). Marriage, as well as the sex act within marriage, has meaning not only because of procreation but also as the expression and fulfilment of a deep union of love. The church has always taught that the marital act retains a meaning and high value even when, through no intervention of ours, conception cannot occur (in the case of sterility, for example).

Lonergan's letter on contraception and the natural law clearly shows how our thinking about marriage has developed and how this new personal data changes our approach to the topic of contraception:

> Besides erroneous Aristotelian biology there has been another factor leading to the change in Catholic theological opinion. It is that sexual intercourse between man and wife both expresses and fosters their mutual love. This is fully

acknowledged in Vatican II and also in *Humanae Vitae*. Aristotle treated not marital intercourse but generation as common to all animals. His oversight has been corrected by contemporary phenomenological inquiry.

While the Encyclical [*Humanae Vitae*] acknowledges the "unitive sense" of marital intercourse, it claims that inseparable from it there is a "procreative sense." This would be easy enough to understand if one still clung to Aristotle's biology. But on contemporary biology, if insemination may be said to be inseparable from normal intercourse, conception cannot be said to be inseparable from insemination. The discharge of two million spermatozoa into the vagina does not mean or intend two million babies. Most of the time it does not mean or intend any babies at all. The relationship of insemination to conception is not the relation of a per se cause to a per se effect. It is a statistical relationship relating a sufficiently long and random series of inseminations with some conceptions.

In my opinion such opinions as are expressed in phrases like "actus per se aptos ad generandum" and "process open to conception" are transitional. They reformulate the Aristotelian position and the resultant Catholic tradition during the interval between the discovery that Aristotelian biology is mistaken and the discovery that marital intercourse of itself, per se, is an expression and sustainer of love with only a statistical relationship to conception.

The examples above all relate to data that Lonergan sees as part of what he calls the object-pole of ethical decision-making. The amassing of this evidence is mostly the concern of others—theologians, historians, biologists, psychologists, sociologists, and so on. In our day, scholars in these fields have expanded our notion of the purposes of marriage, demonstrating that the traditional prohibition of the use of contraceptives reflects outmoded science, setting forth a clearer understanding of the historical origins of the traditional teaching, and providing us with a broader understanding of what constitutes personhood. All of this evidence needs to be considered in critical and authentic ethical decision-making. Of course, because ethical judgments are intrinsically conditioned by the character of the data on which they are based, they are necessarily open to continual refinement and even revision.

Subject-Pole in Ethical Decision-Making

As a Roman Catholic philosopher and theologian, Bernard Lonergan's main interest in ethics centers around the subject-pole; what am I going to do with the complex of data relating to the ethical question at hand (in our example, the morality of artificial birth control). Ethical decision making is not just conditioned by the character of the data *out there* but it is also conditioned by the character of the person making the decision, by the person's authenticity or unauthenticity.

Here one's personal circumstances and experience, one's stage of development, and one's biases loom as significant factors influencing ethical decision-making. This issue of authenticity is twofold: there is what Lonergan calls the "minor authenticity" of subjects with respect to the tradition that has nourished them and the "major authenticity" that justifies or condemns the tradition itself.

Major authenticity is an ongoing struggle. Self appropriation of the generalized empirical method involves paying attention to our experiencing, understanding, and judging but paying attention as well to our *inattention* to certain kinds of data and our personal, cultural, gender, and religious biases. Thus, at times we make mistakes and arrive at judgments informed more by inattention and bias than a real concern for truth and thereupon make decisions that are poorly informed or uninformed. Self-appropriation is concerned with understanding understanding but also is "a campaign against the flight from understanding" (Lonergan, *Insight*, 7). Authentic self-appropriation involves a healthy degree of scepticism and critical knowledge of oneself. "The point," says Lonergan in the Introduction to *Insight*, "is to become able to discriminate with ease and from personal conviction between one's purely intellectual activities and the manifold of other, 'existential' concerns that invade and mix and blend with the operations of intellect to render it ambivalent and its pronouncements ambiguous" (14). Self-appropriation, exercised in this way, produces a truly authentic person. The truth or falsity of one's ethical judgments and decisions "has its criterion in the authenticity or the lack of authenticity of the subject's being" (Lonergan, *Method*, 37).

There is, therefore, a dual creation in our knowing and doing; we not only create objects, we create ourselves (i.e., form character). This critical juncture in our increasing autonomy is where we discover in ourselves and for ourselves that it is ultimately up to ourselves to determine who we are to be (Lonergan, *Third Collection*, 230). Lonergan refers to this appreciation as the "existential moment," "the realization that one not only chooses between courses of action but also thereby makes oneself an authentic human being or an unauthentic one" (Lonergan, *Method*, 38).

Authenticity, then, involves more than just *knowing* the truth; it is knowledge of truth as oriented towards decision for action, towards *doing* the truth and deciding to live that way as a matter of routine. This is a tall order and for Lonergan only possible when we have been "grasped by ultimate concern" (God, for believers). For Christians this "fated acceptance of a vocation to holiness" (*Method*, 240) is the experience of God's love having been "poured into our hearts through the Holy Spirit that has been given to us" (Romans 5:5).

The path to authenticity, however, is not an easy one and many choose to live unauthentic lives; others "authentically realize unauthenticity." Lonergan explains this, perhaps puzzling phraseology, very well:

> divers men can ask themselves whether or not they are genuine Catholics or Protestants, Muslims or Buddhists, Platonists or Aristotelians, Kantians or Hegelians, artists or scientists, and so forth. Now they may answer that they are, and their answer may be correct. But they can also answer affirmatively and still be mistaken. In that case . . . what I am is one thing, what a genuine Christian or Buddhist is, is another, and I am unaware of the difference. My unawareness is unexpressed. I have no language to express what I am, so I use the language of the tradition I unauthentically appropriate, and thereby I devaluate, distort, water down, corrupt that language.
>
> Such devaluation, distortion, corruption may occur only in scattered individuals. But it may occur on a more massive scale, and then the words are repeated, but the meaning is gone. The chair was still the chair of Moses, but it was occupied by the scribes and Pharisees. The theology was still scholastic, but the scholasticism was decadent. The religious order still read out the rules, but one wonders whether the home fires were still burning. The sacred name of science may still be invoked but . . . all significant scientific ideals can vanish to be replaced by the conventions of a clique. So the unauthenticity of individuals becomes the unauthenticity of a tradition. Then, in the measure a subject takes the tradition, as it exists, for his standard, in that measure he can do no more than authentically realize unauthenticity." (Lonergan, *Method*, 80)

Returning to a concrete consideration of the inner, subject-pole, of our contraception example, there are several possibilities. An adult Catholic might uncritically appropriate the traditional church teaching on contraception and not even think of the possibility that it might be flawed. And their efforts to live in accord with the teaching may evoke heroic sacrifices. Clearly, their choice is authentic but, as we have seen in our discussion of the factual data *out there* which comes from a variety of disciplines (ranging from theology to biology), there are reasons to question the authenticity of the teaching being so authentically appropriated. In terms of Lonergan's understanding of human development as proceeding in two ways, this individual is uncritically accepting what has been handed *down* by papal authority. Alternatively a Catholic might make a decision to use artificial means of birth control based largely on personal needs and desires, with little or no reference to church teaching or any other pertinent data; choosing to ignore the transcendental imperative to decide *responsibly*, thereby living unauthentically.

There is another way Catholics have made the inner subject-pole decision about the use of artificial contraception. It is the path of critical realism trod by Bernard Lonergan in his letter on contraception and the natural law. Bernard Lonergan's own life and career, in fact, can be interpreted as the journey of a person *out of* the absolutism in which he was nurtured and *into* modern scientific and historical consciousness (Lonergan, *Second Collection*, 210). One statement of Lonergan that I often quote reflects this view that one can preserve the best of the old tradition and at the same time be open to "new learning." Referring to our modern tendency to "brush aside the old questions of cognitional theory, epistemology, [and] metaphysics," Lonergan said, "I have no doubt, I never did doubt, that the old answers were defective" (*Second Collection*, 86). Note the balance (reflecting the two ways of human development) in this statement; it is not that we have traditionally asked the wrong *questions* (classical science and much that calls itself philosophy today says we did) but that the traditional way of answering them did not take into account advances (largely in terms of historical consciousness and contemporary scientific approaches) that have been made since the classical answers were carved in stone. It is possible to critically and authentically evaluate the data from theology, biology and the historical and human sciences which give rise to questions about the traditional approach to contraception and, in good conscience, make an informed ethical choice not fully in conformity with the official teachings of the church on this matter of artificial conception.[9] Lonergan is quick to point out, however, that such authenticity is never an easy nor a permanent, once and for all, achievement but a daily struggle:

> Human authenticity is not some pure quality, some serene freedom from all oversights, all misunderstandings, all mistakes, all sins. Rather it consists in a withdrawal from unauthenticity, and the withdrawal is never a permanent achievement. It is ever precarious, ever to be achieved afresh, ever in great part a matter of uncovering still more oversights, acknowledging still further failures to understand, correcting still more mistakes, repenting more and more deeply hidden sins. (Lonergan, *Method*, 252)

When we have begun the process of self-constitution from a reflective, critical stance on the responsible level of consciousness, Lonergan asserts, we have come to a critical turning point in our lives—the point at which *spiritual* development, properly speaking, begins. Practical reflection moves us from the realm of fact into that of *value* when we deliberate about the goodness of a possible course of action and right action moves us towards community, towards being-in-love.

Conclusion

Bernard Lonergan has been acclaimed as one of the greatest thinkers of the twentieth century, a man "whose shadow has already fallen far into the next century." *Insight* is routinely referred to as one of the most important works to be published in the world in this century. He is credited with having "closed a seven century gap in Catholic thought."[10]

Lonergan wrote that he had spent eleven years of his life "reaching up to the mind of Aquinas" and once said that he did not think he had succeeded in climbing more than halfway up the mountain of Aquinas' achievements (Lonergan, *Insight*, 769). In my view, we are not even halfway up the mountain of Lonergan's achievement and more than a decade after his death his thought still points us towards an intellectual and moral self-transcendence that we have yet to fully embrace.

Notes

1. Contraception is chosen as our example because it is a topic on which Lonergan commented in an extant letter.

2. It is important to point out here that many Catholics who choose to use artificial birth control recognize Pope Paul VI's genuine pastoral concern for the faithful and affirm the major themes of *Humanae Vitae*. In fact, it is in the agony of trying to reconcile the need to express conjugal love and responsible parenthood that artificial birth control becomes an option.

3. Taken together, the first two levels represent *thinking*, not knowing. Our understanding of the world can be mistaken; it is because we can *mis*understand that a third level, judgment, is needed for knowledge. The level of judgment is where we determine how much of our thinking is correct (Lonergan, *Second Collection*, 31).

4. We don't go on, or at least can't *satisfactorily* go on, until the goal of a given level has been reached. So, every question for reflection presupposes that we have arrived at an answer to a question for intelligence; every question requiring deliberation and decision presupposes that we have answered 'yes' or 'no' to the reflective question, 'Is our understanding of the data correct?' According to Lonergan, deliberation about what action to take sublates and unifies knowing and feeling. It is the context for the whole knowing project; we want to know in order to act responsibly.

5. You may be troubled by human "subjectivity" clearly rearing its head here. Lonergan's claim is that there is a subjective component to *all* knowing and, far from making our knowing suspect, subjectivity is integral to the correct unfolding of the knowing process. In fact, Lonergan argues

that *all* knowing *is* subjective and in an often quoted phrase points out that "genuine objectivity is the fruit of authentic subjectivity. It is to be attained only by attaining authentic subjectivity" (Lonergan, *Method*, 292). As a simple illustration of what Lonergan means by this significant but perhaps enigmatic expression, consider an x-ray. Knowing what an x-ray means is certainly more than just *looking* at shades of light and dark on a sheet of plastic. A radiologist practicing his/her craft *knows* how to interpret (understand) these shadows and to judge that a certain tiny line on the film *means* that the patient has a fractured rib. The radiologist's trained subjectivity arrives at an objectivity that I, by *looking* at the x-ray, cannot reach. Knowing is not just taking a good look; knowing is an interlocking process of attending (sensing, perceiving, and imagining), understanding (inquiring, gaining insight, and formulating), reflecting and judging.

6. Human freedom lies in the *imperative* (not necessary) quality of human consciousness. We are free by our very constitution as human persons. Freedom is always exercised in a matrix of human relationship; in community because we human beings have a "primordial sympathy for one another," Lonergan suggests in *Insight*. We do not live with one another as in an ant hill but in relationship, with feelings and commitments. In community there is a tension between our "primordial sympathy for one another" and the practical needs we have and tasks to be done; between inter-subjectivity and the practical. There can be great lovey-dovey inter-subjectivity but nothing is getting done or the task may be getting done but there is no community. Society should offer both; a healthy social order is one that reflects a balance between inter-subjectivity and the practical.

7. By this Lonergan means that in order to disprove what he is saying you would necessarily have to appeal to a *judgment* you have made that your *understanding* of a particular set of *data* is correct; in other words, you would *necessarily* have to use the process to disprove the process and so Lonergan concludes that "the possibility of a revision presupposes this analysis" (Lonergan, *Understanding and Being*, 143).

8. Letter of Bernard Lonergan on contraception and the natural law (dated September 6, 1968), edited by Frederick E. Crowe and Robert M. Doran and reprinted in the *Lonergan Studies Newsletter*, vol. 11, no. 1 (March, 1990), 7.

9. The teaching of *Humanae Vitae* on the immorality of artificial birth control cannot justifiably be considered as infallibly taught. In fact, as the contents of the encyclical were outlined to the press in 1968, a Vatican spokesperson said twice that it was *not* an infallible statement.

10. *Dictionary of Jesuit Biography: Ministry to English Canada 1842–1987*, 191.

Works Cited

Catechism of the Catholic Church. 1994. Ottawa: Canadian Conference of Catholic Bishops.

Crowe, Frederick E. 1989. *Appropriating the Lonergan Idea.* Edited by Michael Vertin. Washington, DC: The Catholic University of America Press.

————. 1980. *The Lonergan Enterprise* Cambridge, MA: Cowley Publications.

Dictionary of Jesuit Biography: Ministry to English Canada 1842–1987. 1991. Toronto: Canadian Institute of Jesuit Sources, 191.

Flannery, Austin, ed. 1988. *Vatican Council II: The Conciliar and Post Conciliar Documents.* Vol. 1. Northport, NY: Costello Publishing Company.

Gregson, Vernon, ed. 1988. *The Desires of the Human Heart: An Introduction to the Theology of Bernard Lonergan.* Mahwah, NJ: Paulist Press.

Liddy, Richard M. 1993. *Transforming Light: Intellectual Conversion in the Early Lonergan.* Collegeville, MN: The Liturgical Press.

Lonergan, Bernard. 1993. *Topics in Education.* Vol. 10 of the *Collected Works of Bernard Lonergan.* Edited by Frederick E. Crowe and Robert M. Doran, revising and augmenting the unpublished text prepared by James Quinn and John Quinn. Toronto: University of Toronto Press. These lectures were delivered at Xavier University, Cincinnati, in August, 1959.

————. 1992. *Insight: A Study of Human Understanding.* Vol. 3 of the *Collected Works of Bernard Lonergan.* Edited by Frederick E. Crowe and Robert M. Doran. Toronto: University of Toronto Press. *Insight* was first published in 1957.

————. 1990. *Method in Theology.* Toronto: University of Toronto Press for Lonergan Research Institute. *Method in Theology* was first published in 1972.

————. 1990. *Understanding and Being.* Vol. 5 of the *Collected Works of Bernard Lonergan.* Edited by Elizabeth A. Morelli and Mark D. Morelli; revised and augmented by Frederick E. Crowe with the collaboration of Elizabeth A. Morelli, Mark D. Morelli, Robert M. Doran, and Thomas V. Daly. Toronto: University of Toronto Press. *Understanding and Being,* the Halifax Lectures on *Insight,* was first published in 1980.

————. 1988. *Collection.* Vol. 4 of the *Collected Works of Bernard Lonergan.* Edited by Frederick E. Crowe and Robert M. Doran. Toronto: University of Toronto Press. *Collection* was first published in 1967.

————. 1985. *A Third Collection: Papers by Bernard J. F. Lonergan, S.J.* Edited by Frederick E. Crowe, S.J. New York: Paulist Press.

————. "Questionnaire on Philosophy," *Method: Journal of Lonergan Studies* 2, no. 2 (October 1984): 1–35.

————. 1974. *A Second Collection.* Edited by William F. J. Ryan and Bernard J. Tyrrell. Philadelphia: The Westminster Press.

Lonergan Research Institute *Bulletin,* nos. 4–6, November 1989–1991. Toronto: Lonergan Research Institute.

Meynell, Hugo A. 1991. *An Introduction to the Philosophy of Bernard Lonergan.* Toronto: University of Toronto Press.

Pascal, Blaise. 1966. *Pensées.* Translated by A. J. Krailsheimer. London: Penguin Books. *Pensées* was first published soon after Pascal's death in 1662.

Vertin, Michael. 1994. "Lonergan on Consciousness: Is There a Fifth Level?," *Method: Journal of Lonergan Studies* 12, no. 2: 1–36.

Scriptural quotations are from *The New Revised Standard Version*, 1989.

Chapter 8

Gender Hierarchy and Ethics in Islamic Thought

Sheila McDonough

As Muslims are going through the processes of adapting their traditional patterns of family and community life under the pressures of industrialization, the issues related to gender hierarchy are much discussed and disputed among them. The increase of literacy, which gives access to the Qur'an and Islamic history, encourages the dissemination of knowledge to ordinary Muslims about their long and complex cumulative tradition. Many now read and study the Qur'an for themselves, which was, of course, not the case in the Muslim Middle Ages.

The differences of opinion among present day Muslims on these issues spring from different readings of the scripture and of the history of the legal institutions of the Muslim past. All the parties disputing the issues use traditional materials to support their ideas, but they select different aspects of the complex Muslim past to buttress their claims. They all quote the Qur'an, the practice of the Prophet and his Companions, and the jurisprudence of the medieval religious law, *fiqh*. But they do this from different perspectives, and they arrive at different conclusions.

It is important to view these disputes as on-going processes in which issues change, emphases change, and people change. The adaptation of traditional Muslim values to contemporary needs is a complex process. In contemporary Muslim nations, laws have been changing in response to public pressure, and will no doubt continue to do so. The interpretation given to the Muslim past is an important factor in the attitudes to changing and adapting the laws. Further, the degree of education possessed by both male and female citizens is an important factor, as is the role of the press and other sources of information available to citizens.

It is also important to recognize that change is not a matter of Muslim societies simply adapting to western models over the course of time. There are over a billion Muslims in the world now, some of them members of rapidly developing economies such as Malaysia and Indonesia. Many of them envision new forms of Islamic society developing which they think may manifest better forms of social and economic justice than are present in any contemporary western societies. Many Muslims think that Islam is going to be the dominant religion of the future.

With respect to gender, certain issues are not in dispute and others are. What is not disputed is that males and females are created by God and expected to live their lives in expectation of a final meeting with God at the Judgment Day. Men and women have the same religious obligations in terms of the duty to pray five times a day, fast for a month, give alms, witness to the unity of God, and go on pilgrimage to Mecca once in a lifetime if possible. Women and men are responsible adults, and each person will have to answer to his/her creator for the use that has been made of the life that was given.

The year one for Muslims was 622 CE, the year the new Muslim community left their home town of Mecca because of persecution, and established a new way of life in the neighboring city of Medina. Acceptance of the revelation which had come through the Prophet Muhammad meant, for those who became believers, severe conflict with their own people in Mecca, and exile to a new place and a new way of life. Approximately seventy persons went into exile in this way and formed the nucleus of the new pattern of existence which became known as Islam. Now after 1300 years, there are over a billion Muslims in the world, settled everywhere from East Asia to North America.

The original conflict with the citizens of Mecca arose because the new revelation, the Qur'an, insisted on the abolition of idolatry, and the regulation of commerce by forbidding usury. The Meccans vigorously defended their traditional religious and business practices, and three times tried to destroy the new Muslim community in Medina. Not long before the death of the Prophet Muhammad, his opponents in Mecca were finally overcome, and the Muslims returned to their native city, destroyed the idols of the pre-Islamic Arabs and began the development of their new mode of life.

We have available to us several lives of the Prophet Muhammad and his companions which were written within 150 years of his death in 632 CE. This material is something like the *Acts of the Apostles* in the Christian scriptures in that it tells us how the community has remembered the founding events of the tradition. There are three references to the Prophet's first wife, Khadija, in the classical life of the Prophet, written by Ibn Ishaq. She is in many respects a role model for later Muslim women. The first reference is about their marriage which took place before Muhammad began to receive Revelation.

> Khadija was a merchant woman of dignity and wealth. She used to hire men to carry merchandise outside the country on a profit-sharing basis, for Quraysh were a people given to commerce. Now when she heard about the Prophet's truthfulness, trustworthiness, and honorable character, she sent for him and proposed that he should take her goods to Syria and trade with them, while she would pay him more than she paid others. . . . The Apostle of God accepted the proposal . . . and set out for Syria. . . .
>
> Now Khadija at that time was the best born woman in Quraysh, of the greatest dignity and, too, the richest. . . . The Apostle of God . . . married her. (Guillaume, *The Life of Muhammad*, 82 & 83)

The second reference is to the fact that, when Revelation first came to the Prophet Muhammad, he was very distressed. Khadija took firm action, consulting her cousin who was a Christian, and assuring the Prophet that his experience was genuine. The report says that after the experience of Revelation the Prophet was confused about the experience. Khadija assured him the experience had not been a delusion. She said:

> 'God would not treat you thus since he knows your truthfulness, your great trustworthiness, and your fine character, and your kindness. This cannot be, my dear, perhaps you did see something.' 'Yes, I did, I said.' Then I told her of what I had seen; and she said, 'Rejoice, O son of my uncle, and be of good heart. Verily, by Him in whose hand is Khadija's soul, I have hope that thou will be the prophet of his people. (Guillaume, *The Life of Muhammad*, 106–107)

Muhammad is thus the first of the believers, and Khadija the second. Her intervention at this point is understood to have played a significant role in assuring the Prophet of the authenticity of his experience. The final reference to her is about her death, where it is said that she had been a faithful support to the Prophet and that he had told her all his troubles (Guillaume, 191). The image of Khadija is very important for Muslim women. As an exemplar of Muslim piety, she is seen as one who exhibited strength of character, and resourcefulness and energy in her activities in the spread of the new religion. The Prophet Muhammad did not marry anyone else during her lifetime.

The experience of the first Muslim community meant that the first women to accept the revelation entered into conflict with their existing culture, often involving persecution by their families, and had to risk much in order to take part in the life of the new community. It took courage and commitment from women, as well as from men, to break with the patterns of the past in this way and to enter into the adventure of creating new forms of social organization. The community still honors the names of these original women believers much as Christians honor the names of the women who upheld Christian values in the context of Roman paganism in the first Christian centuries.[1]

Acceptance of the new revelation meant response to the Qur'anic affirmation of the existence of the one God, Creator of all that exists, and Final Judge of all human beings. The first Muslim women who accepted this message affirmed as responsible adults that they would bear witness to the one God, and acknowledge the prophethood of Muhammad. The Qur'an addresses women specifically as adults responsible as individuals for accepting the imperatives to live in expectation of final judgment from God.

> For Muslim men and women, for believing men and women, for devout men and women, for true men and women, for men and women who are patient and constant, for men and women who humble themselves, for men and women who give in charity, for men and women who fast [and deny themselves], for men and women who guard their chastity, and for men and women who engage much in God's praise,—for them God has prepared forgiveness and great reward. 33:35 [2]

God is as close as the vein of the throat (50:16), knows the hearts of all persons (42:20–25), and is the transcendent source of life and power (40:65–70). The woman's acceptance of God as Creator and final Judge was, and is, personal; ultimately she is responsible to God alone. There are no priests, sacraments, or mediators between God and humans according to the Qur'an.

After the successes of Muslim expansion in the first Islamic century—during which new Muslim communities were established across North Africa, into Spain, and across the Middle East into India—the community settled down to develop political, social and economic patterns of existence based on the revelation. After about two hundred years, those who are known as the scholar-jurists (*ulama*) worked out a system of interpreting the revelation. They had collected fragments of oral traditions as to what the Prophet and his early companions had said and done (*Hadith*). Once these collections of *Hadith* were written down, in the middle of the ninth century, a method of systematic thinking about legal issues in the light of revelation was devised. *Usul al Fiqh* means principles of jurisprudence. The word *Shariah* means the divine law in the abstract, namely how human life is to be lived. The concrete written source of the abstract ideal is *fiqh*, jurisprudence (Esposito, *Women in Muslin Family Law*, 103).

The *fiqh* books consist of the collections of writings of various schools of jurisprudence and convey the opinions of legal scholars on matters of religious law. There are differences among the major schools of Sunni jurisprudence, and between the Sunni schools and the Shia ones. The institutions of *madrassas* (seminaries) came into existence in the tenth century, namely about three hundred years after the founding events of the tradition, to train the *ulama* using the Qur'an, the written *Hadith*, and the books of jurisprudence as the source of the training. This method of training *ulama* has remained largely the same until the present. A court system functioned in the Muslim middle ages; the judges (*qadis*) were usually trained in the *madrassas*. There were also other forms of law operative in the Muslim middle ages. What is known as *Siyasa Shariah*, political law, represented the laws made by the will of the rulers. This form of law was often not codified and changed from regime to regime.

In the modern world, legislatures in Muslim countries have been gradually adapting the medieval legal codes. The process of adaptation is based on the ideas of public good. The legislatures adapt the medieval codes in the light of what seems reasonable and in the public good. *Ijtihad* is the technical term for exercising reason in the establishment of law.[3] Modernity in the Islamic world basically dates from the French revolution and from the shock occasioned by Napoleon's invasion of Egypt. Changes began to occur throughout the nineteenth century.[4] The codification of law has been one of the major new developments. In the twentieth century, particularly after the end of imperialist domination following World War II, elected legislatures have been at work developing new legal codes in all major Muslim nations.

With respect to gender issues, the male scholar-jurists (*ulama*), trained by the curriculum of the medieval *madrassas*, assumed that the desirable patterns of family and social existence for Muslims required separation of male and female in family and social life, and stressed the authority of the male as head of the family. The separation of male and female is understood in medieval Muslim thought as necessary for the protection of the female. Women are not to leave their homes unless protected by male escorts, and are not to appear in immodest dress in public situations. Generally, the medieval pattern was that female existence was relatively restricted to the home, where social intercourse was mainly between females. The males were the ones who interacted with the world outside the home.[5]

In the modern period, the differences between Muslims on issues of gender hierarchy are based primarily on different opinions as to how much authority should be given to the opinions of the scholar-jurists. The more conservative think of the opinions of these scholar-jurists as indicating a sort of a-historical truth—an essential Islam which has been and always will be the same. Those who differ, see the mental attitudes of the scholar-jurists as products of a particular kind of intellectual training—*madrassa* education—which was shaped consciously and unconsciously by the assumptions about gender which were implicit in the curriculum of these institutions. Those assumptions are said to reflect the gender characteristics of the type of society which existed in the ninth century in the Muslim world.

One Muslim woman scholar, Leila Ahmed, argues that the fundamental Qur'anic imperative to equality before God operated within Islamic history from generation to generation to stimulate Muslims to work for more adequate expressions of social justice in their cultural institutions. She maintains that Muslims hear two voices from their past; one is the ethical voice of the Qur'an advocating equality and justice, and the other is the patriarchal voice of the established form of legal reasoning on gender issues, *fiqh*. She argues that the ninth century scholars who worked out the written codes of religious law were, consciously and unconsciously, shaped by the presuppositions of the cultural system to which they belonged, the Abbasid Empire, (750–1258 CE).[6]

This Empire, centered in Baghdad, was run by Muslims following the models of many other ancient Empires. Thus the Abbasid Caliphs, Muslim heads of state, in fact lived according to the pattern of many pre-Islamic monarchs. From this perspective, the emphasis on patriarchal control over women can be regarded as a largely pre-Islamic practice which entered into Muslim life after the spread of Islam throughout the Middle East and across North Africa and Spain in the seventh and eighth centuries.

The issues in dispute among Muslims in the twentieth century include questions as to how much authority the medieval codes of jurisprudence should exercise over modern Muslims. There is also an old and continuing dispute between Muslim philosophers and jurists as to which of them is better qualified to deal with fundamental ethical issues.[7] The modern issues include recognition of the functioning of the cumulative tradition. In reality, most of those who claim to accept the authority of the medieval codes of jurisprudence do in fact ignore much medieval material that is no longer relevant, such as instructions about dealing with slaves. However, gender hierarchy remains still an urgent and much disputed issue, specifically with respect to the authority of the husband over his wife, to the issue of the head-covering (*hijab*), and to the separation of the sexes in public life. Writers advocating the continuance of the authority of the husband, the *hijab*, and the separation of the sexes tend to do so not only on the basis of their selections of authoritative voices from the Muslim past, but also on the basis of what is alleged to be natural and healthy for a harmonious society.

The first point to make about this latter form of rhetoric is that much of it is attractive and effective for the audience for whom it is written, namely, contemporary Muslim men and women with some degree of education, persons involved in social change, yet intimidated and threatened by what seems to them the breakdown of family life and sensible living in western societies. One finds small books and pamphlets about Muslim marriage and family life in every part of the Muslim world. This literature is often distributed in mosques. Many sermons are preached at the Friday noon prayers on these subjects. Many western converts to Islam are attracted by this Muslim vision of the family. This rhetoric is primarily future oriented in that it is criticizing what are conceived to be evils of the modern West in order to advocate and to try to create a better society.

One of the most popular books on Muslim ethics was written by a scholar, Hammudah Abd al Ati, who came in the fifties from the Azhar University in Cairo to the Institute of Islamic Studies at McGill; he subsequently served as an Imam of the first mosque in Canada, the al-Rashid Mosque in Edmonton. His book *Islam in Focus* was first published from that mosque while he was serving there in the sixties. He wrote as follows about marriage and gender hierarchy.

> Whatever meanings people assign to marriage, Islam views it as a strong bond. . . . It is a commitment to life itself, to society, and to the dignified meaningful survival of the human race. . . . To paraphrase some Qur'anic verses, the call is addressed to mankind to be dutiful to God, Who created them from a single soul, (4:1). . . . And it is a sign of God that He has created for men, of themselves, mates to seek in their company peace and tranquillity and has set between them mutual love and mercy. Surely, in that are signs for those who contemplate (30:21). Even at the most trying times of married life, and in the midst of legal disputes and litigation, the Qur'an reminds the parties of God's law; it commands them to be kind to one another, truly charitable toward one another, and above all dutiful to God. . . .
>
> The role of the husband evolves around the moral principle that it is his solemn duty to God to treat his wife with kindness, honor and patience. . . . (Qur'an 2:229–32, 4:19) The role of the wife is summarized in the verse that women have rights even as they have duties, according to what is equitable; but men have a decree over them (2:228). This decree is usually interpreted by Muslim scholars in conjunction with another passage which states, among other things, that men are trustees, guardians and protectors of women because God has made some of them excel others and because they expend of their means.
> (Abd al Ati, *Islam in Focus*, 117)

> Men are the protectors and maintainers of women because God has given the one more (strength) than the other, and because they support them from their means. Therefore the righteous women are devoutly obedient. (4:34)

Hammudah Abd al Ati says that the degree of authority given to the male may be what sociologists call 'instrumental leadership' or external authority in the household due to the division of labor and role differentiation. He says it does not mean any categorical discrimination or superiority of one to the other.

A somewhat different interpretation of the same Qur'anic passage is given by a Muslim woman scholar who has recently published a commentary on the Qur'an. One issue is whether or not the male was created first, and the female created from him, as Hammudah Abd al Ati and the scholar-jurists before him have assumed. From this male angle, woman exists to help man; her obedience is therefore reasonable. The Qur'anic passage in question reads: "O mankind! reverence your Guardian-Lord, who created you from a single Person, created, of like nature, his mate, and from them twain scattered (like seeds) countless men and women" (4:1).

Traditional Qur'anic exegesis has usually assumed, perhaps partly under the influence of ideas from Jewish and Christian converts who took the biblical narrative as significant, that this passage meant the male was created first and the female created from him, to be his "help-mate" as the Bible says in Genesis 2:18. However, Amina Wadud-Muhsin argues (partly following Yusuf Ali), that the 'single Person' referred to in this English translation of the Qur'an was not a single male human, but rather some abstract personal soul-stuff—*nafs*—and that male and female came into being at the same time from the *nafs*. This is supported by the fact that many other Qur'anic references indicate that God customarily creates in pairs in all the diverse species he creates (51:49). This point is important because arguments for equality among the sexes have more force if they are legitimated by the view that creation was the same for both. It makes a difference whether or not one thinks that gender hierarchy has an ontological basis, i.e., is founded on the fundamental reality of existence.

Another disputed issue is the interpretation of the passage (4:34) which Hammudah Abd al Ati referred to in discussing male superiority and the need for the wife to be obedient: "Men are (*qawwanmuna ala*) women" (4:34).

Amina Wadud-Muhsin deals as follows with this passage:

Needless to say, this verse covers a great deal more than just preference. This is classically viewed as the single most important verse with regard to the relationship between men and women. . . .

As for the meaning, Pickthall translates this as 'in charge of'. Al Zamakhshari says it means that 'men are in charge of the affairs of woman.' Maududi says 'Men are the managers of the affair of women because Allah has made the one superior to the other. . . .' Azizah al-Hibri [a woman scholar] objects to any translation which implies that men are protectors or maintainers because 'The basic notion here is one of moral guidance and caring' and also because; '. . . only in extreme conditions [for example, insanity] does the Muslim woman lose her right to self-determination'. . . . Yet men have used this passage to exercise absolute authority over women. They also use it to argue for the males's divinely ordained and inherent superiority. . . .

I [Amina Wadud-Muhsin] apply this verse to society at large but not on the basis of inherent superiority of men over women, or of Allah's preference of men over women. Rather, I extend the functional relationship which Sayyid Qutb proposes between the husband and the wife towards the collective good concerning the relationship between men and women in society at large. My main consideration is the responsibility and right of women to bear children . . . . The child-bearing responsibility is of grave importance; human existence depends upon it. . . . For simple balance and justice in creation, and to avoid oppression, his [the males] responsibility must be equally significant to the continuance of the human race. The Qur'an established his responsibility: seeing to it that the woman is not burdened with additional responsibilities which jeopardize that primary demanding responsibility that only she can fulfil.

Ideally, *everything* she needs to fulfil her primary responsibility comfortably should be supplied by society, namely by the male: this means physical protection as well as material sustenance. . . .

All of these issues cannot be resolved if we look narrowly at verse 4:34. Therefore, the Qur'an must eternally be reviewed with regard to human exchange and mutual responsibility between males and females. This verse established an ideal obligation for men with regard to women to create a balanced and shared society. This responsibility is neither biological nor inherent, but it is valuable. . . .

. . . Such an attitude will overcome the competitive and hierarchical thinking which destroys rather than nurtures.[8]

Amina Wadud-Muhsin thus argues that men have a responsibility to help women in terms of pregnancy and child raising by working to create a society which would be as just as possible to women. This is a new way of thinking about the Muslim emphasis on gender responsibilities.

Much contemporary Islamic rhetoric stresses complementary gender roles. The contemporary *hijab*, head scarf, which is now used widely in many Muslim societies might be considered a characteristic symbol of a kind of progressive-conservative Islamic attitude. It has become widely used among Muslims since the 1980's. The *hijab* is very different from the various forms of dress worn in medieval Muslim societies. The latter forms of dress, such as the *chador* and the *burkah*, tended to cover the whole body and often the face as well. The *hijab* covers the hair but leaves the face free. Thus, Muslim women wearing the *hijab* are mobile and are also signaling men to leave them alone.

One of the complexities of the debate is that different persons give different weight to the authority of medieval jurisprudence, but few explicitly imagine returning to all of its ways of thought. The difference between the modern *hijab* and the traditional conservative dress symbolizes a basic difference from the medieval even in apparently conservative Muslim thought. Perhaps one could best envisage these different perspectives by thinking of a totally covered woman (medieval style), a *hijab* wearing modern Muslim woman, and a Muslim woman with an uncovered head. In terms of contemporary voices speaking for Muslim values, the first possibility scarcely exists any more.

The second possibility is extremely active at present. One of the female leaders of the movement generally known as political Islam is Zaynab al Ghazali of Egypt. Political Islam, or Islamist, is a general term for types of modern Muslim organizations with specific political agendas. These groups wish to see the Muslim world modernized and industrialized quickly, but they consider modern western society morally corrupt. They think they are going to build a better future than what presently exists in the West. The rhetoric of these groups stresses moral degradation in the West in terms of child and wife abuse, teen-age pregnancies, single parents, alcoholism and drugs, and a general loss of healthy family life. When flying into Malaysia, an economically prosperous and advanced Muslim country, passengers are warned that the death penalty will be given to any one smuggling drugs into the country. This is just one example of the message that many Muslims intend to do things differently.

In Zaynab al Ghazali's writings, the Islamist position, as summarized by Sherifa Zuhur as follows:

Woman serves her God and her *ummah* [community] through marriage and reproduction. She is a further asset to her community when she affirms her position within the nuclear family. She should value her duties to her husband and children more than her own career or other outside goals. Married life can be a virtuous existence. If she can manage to also serve her movement with her husband's consent, so much the better. Women in traditionally female occupations are not instructed to leave their jobs, but they are also admonished to consider their families their first priority. After all, obstetricians, nurses, secretaries and teachers will be required in an Islamist Egypt as they are in the contemporary system.

Since the family is the basic unit of society, factors that threaten the family must be attacked. Society must not encourage illicit extramarital affairs. Sexual temptation must be controlled through law, the wearing of *hijab*, limitations on mixing of the sexes outside the home, peer pressure, and self-policing.

Women are as responsible as men for the condition of the state of society as a whole, and so they must be included in the political process. The government should consult women as citizens, and their husbands must consult them individually. Their reproductive functions are to be controlled but not terminated. *If* they do not abandon family life, they retain the right to work, to participate in the affairs of the movement and ultimately, then, in the state. (Zuhur, *Revealing Reveiling*, 88)

This discussion indicates that issues of gender hierarchy are being vigorously debated among Muslims. In almost all Muslim countries, women have access to education and the vote, and, as Zaynab al Ghazali indicates, most of them intend to make their voices heard in one way or another. There are also many Muslim women who do not cover their heads, and who consider that they are also devout and serious Muslim persons.

Notes

1. See Marcia K. Hermansen, "The Female Hero in the Islamic Religious Tradition," in *The Annual Review of Women in World Religions Volume II Heroic Women*, edited by Arvind Sharma and Katherine K. Young, 112–142.

2. All references to the Qur'an are taken from Yusuf Ali *The Meaning of the Glorious Qur'an Text and Explanatory Translation* (Muslim Students Association, 1975).

3. For a good discussion of the role of reason in Islamic law see: Mohammad Hashim Kamali, *Principles of Islamic Jurisprudence*, 366–392. See also Noel J. Coulson, *Conflicts and Tensions in Islamic Jurisprudence*.

4. See Niyazi Berkes, *The Rise of Secularism in Turkey*.

5. See Unni Wikan, *Behind the Veil in Arabia: Women in Oman*.

6. See Leila Ahmed, *Gender and Women in Islam*.

7. See Muhsin Mahdi, "Religious Belief and Scientific Belief," in *The American Journal of Islamic Social Sciences*, vol. 2, no. 2: 245–259.

8. See Amina Wadud-Muhsin, *Qur'an and Woman*, 70–74.

Works Cited

Abd al Ati, Hammudah. 1975. *Islam in Focus*. Indianapolis: American Trust Publications.

Ahmed, Leila. 1993. *Women and Gender in Islam: Historical Roots of a Modern Debate*. New Haven, CT: Yale University Press.

Ali, Yusuf. 1975. *The Meaning of the Glorious Qur'an: Text and Explanatory Translation*. Muslim Students Association of the United States and Canada.

Berkes, Niyazi. 1964. *The Development of Secularism in Turkey*. Montreal: McGill University Press.

Coulson, Noel J. 1969. *Conflicts and Tensions in Islamic Jurisprudence*. Chicago: University of Chicago Press.

Esposito, John L. 1982. *Women in Muslim Family Law*. Syracuse, NY: Syracuse University Press.

Guillaume, A., trans. 1970. *The Life of Muhammad: A Translation of Ishaq's Sirat Rasul Allah*. London: Oxford University Press.

Hermansen, Marcia K. 1992. "The Female Hero in the Islamic Religious Tradition." In *The Annual Review of Women in World Religions: Volume II Heroic Women*, edited by Arvind Sharma and Katherine K. Young. Albany: State University of New York Press.

Kamali, Mohammad Hashim. 1991. *Principles of Islamic Jurisprudence*. Cambridge: Islamic Texts Society.

Mahdi, Muhsin. 1994. "Religious Belief and Scientific Belief." *The American Journal of Islamic Social Sciences,* vol. 2, no 2: 245–259.

Wadud-Muhsin, Amina. 1995. *Qur'an and Woman*. London: Oxford University Press.

Wikan, Unni. 1982. *Behind the Veil in Arabia: Women in Oman*. Baltimore: Johns Hopkins University Press.

Zuhur, Sherifa. 1992. *Revealing Reveiling: Islamic Gender Ideology in Contemporary Egypt*. Albany: State University of New York Press.

PART II

CONTEMPORARY CHALLENGES

Chapter 9

Feminist Scholarship: the Challenge to Ethics

Morny Joy

Is reason "masculine?"[1] In Western thought, have the processes and structures associated with the intellect been so dominated by men that many women still regard philosophy as hostile and alien territory? How are imbalances in power that have regulated most social interactions between men and women to be modified? These are just some of the questions that challenge contemporary feminist thinkers when they begin to question the traditional exclusion and/or denigration of women. Does the fault lie in a conscious and deliberate plot organized by a patriarchal system? Is woman a captive of biological processes that predispose her to emotional and domestic preoccupations? Or are "feminine," as are "masculine" characteristics, simply culturally dependent stereotypes that can be revised to suit the needs of a more egalitarian agenda? Feminist responses to these investigations are extremely varied. There is no single program of activity or set of principles that would be acceptable to all women who identify themselves as feminist. Thus, when it comes to trying to describe the contribution of feminist thought to ethics, it is impossible to specify *the* feminist position. There are many different options that feminists of different persuasions—radical, liberal, Marxist, pluralist—support. They are not all compatible. Nonetheless, they are all vitally concerned with changing the role of women as ethical agents, and with revising the standard male-identified orientations of ethical theory.

In this essay I will not attempt a comprehensive overview of feminist ethics and the various allegiances that have emerged—this has been done elsewhere.[2] Instead, I will undertake a selective thematic discussion which will highlight some of the major trends that have become apparent in the last twenty years. Thus, it is not an exhaustive study, as the literature is so vast that this would be impossible.[3]

I will choose relevant texts to illustrate each trend. My aim is to provide references and resources for further research. I will focus my discussion on three principal themes which illustrate diverse approaches to feminist ethics. Each area emphasizes a particular topic which is regarded as crucial to a revision of ethical theory and practice. The primary focus will be the relevance for religious ethics. This is a somewhat idiosyncratic selection, but it has helped me to organize the material in a coherent, if provisional way. It may not be acceptable to everyone, as it is obviously influenced by my particular biases and background,[4] but I hope that it will provide stimulus for further investigation and debate on these controversial topics.

I have designated the three thematic headings as: an ethics and politics of equality; an ethics of feminine difference; an ethics of pluralism. In all of this discussion, it is often difficult to draw the line where secular thought ends and religious ethics begins. Women's experiences regarding issues of goodness, justice, responsibility have been similarly mandated and imposed by both church and state. The madonna/whore complex has been endemic to most moral reflections regarding the status of women. Women are only now beginning to challenge a God made in the image of the male of the species, and attempting to express new insights that fundamentally change the presuppositions of the predominant ethical code.

An Ethics and Politics of Equality

It is a sad and lamentable fact that in the history of Western philosophy and theology, women have been regarded as unworthy of inclusion in the privileged ranks of those who initiate and put into practice decrees of reason.[5] Men have been accorded a superior value and status that has led to women being variously associated with feelings, nature, the body, the private realm, and the aesthetic, insofar as these things are posited as the opposite of and inferior to reason and its sphere of control. Such a phenomenon has had far-reaching effects. As Nancy Tuana observes: "Philosophers' gender assumptions often affect the central categories of their system—their conceptions of rationality, their construals of the nature of morality, their visions of the public realm" (Tuana, *Woman and the History of Philosophy*, 116). While the whole issue of sex and gender and their interrelationship is a highly debated one in contemporary feminist discussions,[6] what is obvious is that traditional thought didn't worry particularly about these distinctions so that, inevitably, gendered "feminine characteristics," such as irrationality, immorality, and emotionality were, for better or worse, regarded as the domain of the female of the species.

With regard to ethics, the basic problem was that women were not considered as capable of being ethical agents who could make autonomous moral decisions. From Aristotle, to Kant, Hegel,[7] and Freud[8]—to mention the most prominent thinkers—women's capacities were downgraded. Even when she was not regarded as intrinsically evil, woman could not be trusted. Pervasive throughout Western thought is also the denigration of women's bodies themselves. Women are denied the integrity of either mind or body—woman's body predisposes her to evil, yet her mind, as if by contamination, does not have the requisite expertise to help control it or to understand and express alternative positive modes of ethical conduct. Women are thus powerless to change the system that so construes them.

Many contemporary women ethicists are outraged by this legacy they have inherited and are adamant that these distortions of woman and of her body must be corrected. At the same time, the myth of the neutral, detached, male agent whose objective decisions have defined and implemented the parameters of rationality, must be exposed.

In the field of Christian ethics, one of the most articulate women who has undertaken this massive task with courage and passion is Beverly Wildung Harrison. Her two principal publications are milestones in the field of feminist ethics. In *Making the Connections*, she states her mandate: "The task of a Christian feminine ethic is to undermine any morality of blind command and replace it with the process of moral reflection that comes from those who respectfully reason together" (Harrison, *Making the Connections*, 41). Harrison is insistent that women are full participants in such discussions and that the refusal to acknowledge the legitimate moral contributions of women has been "not only a historical, logical, and theological error but also a moral failing" (Harrison, *Our Right to Choose*, 7). At the same time, Harrison is aware that rational reflection has for too long subscribed to an ideal of disembodied knowledge, and that this distortion needs to be rectified by an acceptance that "all our knowledge, including our moral knowledge, is body-mediated knowledge" (*Making the Connections*, 13). This relationship mediates not just self-awareness, but also any apprehension of and response to others (13).[9]

As a case-study to develop and illustrate her beliefs, Harrison investigates the issue of abortion. This is a highly emotionally charged and controversial topic, and my intention is not to defend her position.[10] I would like instead to demonstrate how, for Harrison, the abortion debate is crucial for a reevaluation of traditional ethics that, on this subject, still seeks to control women's bodies and sexuality as well as deprive her of moral agency. "The culture of reproduction" (*Our Right to Choose*, 56), while certainly a personal preoccupation of women, is situated within a wider field of women's fertility, the monitoring of which has long been a male prerogative. As Harrison observes, women's fecundity has been related to male exhibitions of "power, virility and wealth" (162). Hence, as contemporary conditions allow women more freedom, there is a frenzied and vituperative campaign to prevent woman from having a vital role in making decisions regarding her reproductive choices. What Harrison graphically conveys concerning this movement is how minimal, in all the theoretical appeals to the sanctity of life, has been the attention to the life situation of the woman who is involved in an act of extreme moral gravity.

> Few even pause to notice that the question of whether to seek an abortion arises concretely within the life of a woman only under specific circumstances— circumstances that are not mere "externals" to the consideration of abortion but are integral to the full meaning of the dilemma . . . The habit of discussing abortion as if it were a "discrete deed" is a way of formulating the abortion issue as a moral question abstracted out of, and hence irrelevant to, the way it arises in women's lives. (Harrison, *Our Right to Choose*, 9)

This attention to the concrete and particular circumstances, however, does not mean that Harrison supports an individualistic, in the sense of a selfish, frame of reference. Harrison is wary of the abstract appeal to rights in the liberal tradition for a number of reasons, but in this context, her reservations have to do with its emphasis on a person as a monadic entity rather than as a member of a community.[11] In its stead, she supports a communitarian ethic where "the moral and religious vision underlying a feminist commitment places deep and realistic concern for basic community at the center" (*Our Right to Choose*, 55). This communal core recognizes the intrinsically social nature of humanity, but also the complex interrelatedness of the social with the biological and the historical dimensions of existence. While responsibility for decision-making is thus contextual, the context is multifaceted and the reverberations are never confined to the personal.

> By virtue of our agency, we are always cocreative participants in reproduction. Culture, society, and history shape this meaning of pregnancy. Therefore, the expression of the human power of procreation never has occurred outside a relational context of human cocreation. (Harrison, *Our Right to Choose*, 102)

A central component of Harrison's project is a revised conception of God, for as she is well aware, within a religious ethical perspective, theological presuppositions are decisive. Divine and transcendent reality, associated with immutable laws, intransigent authority, and absolute power, has been the mouthpiece of misogynistic and condescending sentiments regarding women. In this scheme of things, as subordinate to man, women are not regarded as being made in the image of God. The best they could do, for the greater part of human history, was to submit to the will of males who believed that they alone could interpret divine decrees.

Unsurprisingly, Harrison believes that this image of God is no longer acceptable and that gendered idealizations are inappropriate.

> God is not the "wholly other" projected by patriarchal piety; nor is God the "He" who remains unaffected by the world. God is the proceeding one, a representing power present to us as companion, one who supports, encourages, lures us into activity in relation. We encounter God through relationship with all that nurtures and sustains life. (Harrison, *Our Right to Choose*, 108)

As well as rejecting artificial binaries which estrange and divide, e.g., male/female, mind/body, nature/history, Harrison wants to rethink the transcendent/immanent dichotomy and see them instead as intimately related. She does this by advocating a process model which appreciates God as participant in creation, as supportive of inclusive and reciprocal connections that inform equitable expressions of love and justice.

> In feminist terms, God is not the One who stands remotely in control, but the One who binds us and bids us to deep relationality, resulting in a radical equality motivated by genuine mutuality and interdependence. (Harrison, *Our Right to Choose*, 99)

Harrison's radical revisions of the traditional ethical framework seek to establish the question of abortion as principally a moral issue, though there are inevitably legal and political ramifications.[12] Her arguments are presented against a wider background that views woman as a moral agent in her own right, whose rational capacity has intrinsic worth, and who has the authority to make judgments concerning not just procreation but sexuality itself. Women's bodies remain a battleground, fought over by competing forces that wish to contain and regulate them. From the perspective of an ethics of equality, unless women of all classes and backgrounds are accorded the dignity of ethical subjectivity,[13] ethics will remain a compromised and partisan enterprise, misrepresenting itself as representative of all humanity.

An Ethics of Feminine Difference

There is another group of feminist scholars who, while they are not completely opposed to rationality, have serious reservations about it (or about its applications). For them, reason is regarded as associated with universal principles and appeals to justice that do not respond with sufficient concern to the particulars of actual situations. These feminists invoke "feminine" virtues, such as care, as decisive for a distinctive approach of ethical responsibility. In recent years, in the wake of such books as Carol Gilligan's *In a Different Voice*, Sara Ruddick's *Maternal Thinking* and Nel Noddings' *Caring*, women have passionately debated these issues.[14] There are other feminist scholars who, in turn, see these developments as simply reinforcing established stereotypes regarding "feminine" behavior, or as implying that there are essential "feminine" values that need to be respected.[15] They also allege that the "feminine" significance of these proposals is based on an irreconcilable opposition to "masculine" modes. These critical feminists believe that, rather than reformative, such a program is counter-productive in its effects.

In this essay, I will concentrate on the work of Noddings in that it exemplifies an attempt to build an ethic of caring and love, which ostensibly does not resort to traditional Christian injunctions. And, while Noddings may be compared to Harrison for her emphasis on context, as well as for her insistence on communality or connectedness, Noddings does not want to accord to rationality the same weight that Harrison does. Instead, Noddings will focus on emotional interaction as the source and sustenance of her theory.

> I shall locate the very well-spring of ethical behavior in human affective response. Throughout our discussion of ethicality we shall remain in touch with the affect that gives rise to it. (Noddings, *Caring*, 3)

Quite explicitly, Noddings describes this as the "feminine view" (*Caring*, 3). In expounding this position, Noddings states: "Women can and do give reasons for their acts, but the reasons often point to feelings, needs, impressions, and a sense of personal ideal rather than to universal principles and their application" (3). "Women often define themselves as both persons and agents in terms of their capacity to care" (40). For Noddings, this propensity finds its fullest (and perhaps most fulfilling) exemplification in the role of motherhood, for she believes that mothering elicits the profoundest emotional response.

> I am working deliberately toward criteria that will preserve our deepest and most tender human feelings. The caring of mother for child, of human adult for human

infant, elicits the tenderest feelings in most of us. Indeed, for many women, this feeling of nurturance lies at the very heart of what we assess as good. (Noddings, *Caring*, 87)

Ultimately, it is the feeling of care, rather than reason that, extrapolated from the mother-child relationship, is promoted as the ideal informing all human exchange. At the same time, this type of caring is posited not just as an aspect of the human condition itself, but as that aspect which is regarded as the prototype of goodness. But if such a feeling occurs naturally, how do we become alienated from it? Is it the fault of men and of their less caring rational orientation? And what of women who do not mother? By singling out motherhood as a paradigm for moral goodness, Noddings would initially seem to be both idealizing and naturalizing a selective situation, then asking it to bear an immense burden of moral authority.

Noddings does not address such problematic areas. Her only refinement is to draw a distinction between natural caring and ethical caring. Natural caring is dependent on the ethical in situations where, according to Noddings, human desire is not in accord with the natural impulse. In this case, the duty to care, the "I must," can be summoned by recalling "our best self," i.e., "our best picture of ourselves caring and being cared for" (*Caring*, 80). Such an explanation does not particularly clarify her position, as the innate characteristic to care thus changes to become something of a regulative ideal, which is exactly the type of abstract command that Noddings is attempting to transcend. Questions arise. What ensures that memories of being loved or cared for remain sufficiently vital to stimulate us, against inclination, to care? Can we be compelled to care?

Again, Noddings does not anticipate such queries, but continues to enumerate the further attributes, such as receptivity, relatedness, and reciprocity that she appreciates as necessary components of a relationship of caring. Noddings' arguments, while their intent is not to discredit rationality entirely, nonetheless demonstrate that sentiment is primary.

Instrumental thinking may, of course, enhance caring; that is, I may use my reasoning powers to figure out what to do once I have committed myself to doing something. But clearly, rationality (in its objective form) does not of necessity mark either the initial impulse or the action that is undertaken. (Noddings, *Caring*, 36)

Such a sweeping and challenging statement is born of Noddings conviction that reason, while illuminative, is not sufficiently attuned to the particular, the concrete. And while she does not deny that men may respond emotionally, or that women may avail themselves of reason, Noddings' whole approach promotes the perspective that women have always inevitably lived in accordance with such moral excellence. For Noddings, it is not then a question of women being given equal access to a rational and ethical code, but a revision of the whole ethical enterprise, so that women's purported timeless affinity with affective bonds become instead the proper criteria for ethical evaluation.

There have been a number of criticisms of this position.[16] One major point of dissent is the unproblematized connection made between women and "the feminine." Though feminine characteristics have come to be viewed by many as intrinsically related to women, the argument is made that caring and self-sacrifice are not innate qualities, but a cultural imposition on women. These stereotypes have freed men to follow their pursuits in the public realm, while women, confined to the private, domestic sphere, have been responsible for managing the emotional economy. The critics allege that such an artificial and unjust division, which perpetuates asymmetrical power arrangements, would, if Noddings' theory is accepted, continue to operate to the detriment of women.

Another objection is that motherhood is unrealistically and universally sanitized. Motherhood is not necessarily a joyous experience, nor is care automatically involved. Nancy Scheper-Hughes depicts the life of women in a shanty-town, where mother love or caring is a luxury that these women cannot afford.[17] Such a contrast indicates that the prevalent descriptions of motherhood in the literature of caring reflect only the values of white, educated, middle-class women. A third criticism sees the whole maternal movement as described as positing a false separation between an ethics of rights ("masculine") and an ethics of responsibility/care ("feminine").[18] Other contemporary feminists, however, would assert that this distinction need not be so stark. Some posit different forms of rapprochement between an ethics of rights and an ethics of care.[19]

The challenge of feminist scholarship that results from the ethics of difference debate reflects a constellation of issues that need to be addressed. One area is the perceived anomaly in the deliberations and administration of justice. As it stands, women have been and continue to be largely excluded (both theoretically and practically) from these proceedings. To redress this imbalance, appeals have been made in the language of rights. But advocates of difference are dissatisfied with such appeals as they feel they perpetuate the present system. As such, they reject the "add women and stir" framework of equality as not being sufficiently attentive to other dimensions of women's experience. The proposed ethics of care highlights the qualities that "difference feminists" want to be primary in moral considerations, whether public or private. Yet it is often unclear how reform is to be effected. The present system continues to be rather intractable when it comes to "feminine" values, and ambivalence about whether these values are the prerogative of women only, or should be inculcated in men as well, impedes reform. The ensuing debate has nonetheless brought into prominence contemporary interpretations of the notion of justice, and its relation to care and goodness, and how, from a feminist perspective, the generally accepted definitions are narrow and selective in their applications. In particular, it has brought attention to the engendering of reason and of ethics. Whether this is an artificial and anachronistic interpolation, requiring correction, or whether the balance of values simply needs to be readjusted, is a fiercely debated issue.

An Ethics of Pluralism

An ethics of difference is built on the understanding that women have been classified as "the other" of men. "Otherness," as a term, indicates the category of difference. In certain Western models, such as interpretations of the Hegelian dialectic, otherness has come to indicate an idea or an entity that needs to be eliminated or assimilated. Very rarely has the other been allowed a voice of its own, and the accepted mind set or the mores of the dominant culture has prevailed. Contemporary feminists, as illustrated in the two previous sections, have exalted or attempted to rectify the resultant lack of equivalence in the classification of gendered characteristics. Yet there are other feminists, such as lesbians, who argue that sex and gender are too narrowly construed.[20] There are also women, not of Anglo-European origin, who argue that gender is not the only category of difference; race and class distinctions have also led to spurious and unjust displacements. Such women believe their voices have not been heard in either the ethics of equality or ethics of difference debates, and contest their exclusion in the same way that women have protested their neglect by men. Attention to these other voices, be they lesbian, African-American, Asian-American, or Hispanic has led to further refinements in feminist ethics so as to promote an ethics of pluralism.

María Lugones, who identifies herself as a lesbian Hispanic, is an impassioned advocate not for inclusion, but for a new responsiveness to the voice of other women in all their particularity. Lugones introduces the notion of "world"-traveling, as a mode of interaction that does not reduce the worlds of either participant to a common denominator. Difference is respected.

> The reason why I think that traveling to someone's "world" is a way of identifying with them is because by traveling to their "world" we can understand *what it is to be them and what it is to be ourselves in their eyes.* Only when we

have traveled to each other's "worlds" are we fully subject to each other. (Lugones, "Playfulness," 17)

The accompanying invocation by Lugones of complexity, ambiguity, and diversity are all catch phrases of the postmodern movement,[21] (even if she never uses the word), and introduce the issue of relativism. There is a resemblance between Lugones' "world"-traveling and Rosi Braidotti's postmodern style of a (feminist) nomadism which flourishes in intersections and transitions, rather than seeking a permanent definition or form of identity. As a strategy, it seeks to disrupt misuse of power—either personal or political—but it resists confinement to any normative designation.

> The feminist postmodernist task is to figure out how to respect cultural diversity without falling into relativism or political despair. Relativism is a pitfall in that it erodes the grounds for possible interalliances or political coalitions. The challenge for feminist nomads in particular is how to conjugate the multilayered, multi cultural perspective, with responsibility for and accountability to their gender. (Braidotti, *Nomadic Subjects*, 31–32)

The charge usually leveled at such an approach is that it is incapable of taking an ethical stand, for by disputing universal determinations, it renders notions of goodness and of justice ineffective. What Braidotti would argue is that postmodern feminism is alert to the abuses of power, particularly the marginalizations and disenfranchisements of women that still occur while lip service is being paid to such ideals as justice. But in the eyes of scholars such as Lugones, postmodernism will remain simply a further tool of oppression and injustice unless it can also undermine the interlocking chains of racism with sexism that are mutually reinforcing.

There are, however other readings of postmodernism that use it in a constructive mode, believing that though it is wary of the myth of modernity and "of the development of society in accordance with a universal and transcendent reason, it [still] works comfortably with reasons. Thereby it is not placed outside rationalism" (Yeatman, *Postmodern Revisionings*, 9). Though rationalism is stressed, I believe that the emphasis here is on differing forms of reason. The type of dominant, analytic, impersonal reasoning associated with the dispassionate, deontological, and utilitarian ethical formulas of the Enlightenment give way to more communally-based and context sensitive responses. This does not necessarily imply an indiscriminate relativism, as the dialogue involved acknowledges the importance of standards, though these do not derive from a single, intransigent source. The resultant negotiations cannot but still be influenced by the traditional Western heritage, though other (including non-Western) perspectives are respected as also providing ethical guidelines. Such contributions have not always been welcome in the monolithic facade of logical argument, impartial rules and principles that have been the mainstay of Western ethical dogmatism.

One recent work in Christian ethics that is exemplary in its deployment of both postmodern categories and reason, without succumbing to the extremes of either, is Marilyn Legge's, *The Grace of Difference: A Canadian Feminist Theological Ethic*. Legge writes as one animated by a Christian theology of liberation which "assumes that our primary transformations as persons come from *conversion and commitment to the other*, to those deemed insignificant and pushed to the margin of our society and to marginal and oppressed peoples of the world" (Legge, *The Grace of Difference*, 12). Thus, though her focus is women, there is solidarity with all those who are relegated to the status of the other, and who thereby suffer unjustly. Legge's focus is both expansive and responsive to the present conservative social climate's exclusions:

> The "margin," as we shall see, is not a static category. It is meant to indicate some tendencies that are structurally determined by nation, region, ethnicity, age, sexuality, race, gender, and class, but which cannot be reduced to these. In today's political climate "the others" include people of color, homosexuals, the poor, feminists, socialists, and even left-liberals. (Legge, *The Grace of Difference*, 25)

What is remarkable here, in the formulation of a feminist ethics, is the range of concern that this ethics takes into account, without presuming to speak on anyone's behalf. This is particularly true regarding the importance of hearing the divergent voices of women (*The Grace of Difference*, 98–99). There is also the awareness that no false generalizations, of either a theoretical or a practical nature, should be made:

> While the structures of race, class, culture, and gender have distinctive historical manifestations and combinations, the point is to construe their relevance for the best possible strategies of social change, and not to be dogmatic about assigning timeless priority to one or another . . . The point is not to deny that equal pay and shared domestic work are common goods; rather . . . race, class, and gender take different tolls on different women, and thus demand different strategies for transformation. (Legge, *The Grace of Difference*, 98–99)[22]

Legge's discussions of the works of the womanist theologians and ethicists, Katie Cannon and Dolores Williams,[23] other African-Americans such as Diane

Brand, Bell Hooks, and Audre Lorde, as well as with women theologians from Asia and South America, are examples of an attentive listening that does not presuppose familiarity, nor impose distortions.[24] The ethical task is one of solidarity, rather than a uniform recipe for resistance. But Legge is nonetheless clear that the primary impetus is one of achieving justice, though again, this can only be introduced in concrete instances as an answer to specific unjust impositions of power.

> Unless we learn to identify the location of power in class, race and culture as well as sex/gender in the routines of everyday life, we will circumvent tackling the problem of the nature of power and the ways in which it is held by some rather than others. (Legge, *The Grace of Difference*, 131)

Legge's goal is for women to achieve well-being in personal and public spheres, (*The Grace of Difference*, 131) but such well-being can only occur when there is justice and right relations. Though these values could coincide with secular criteria, for Legge they are grounded in a theological orientation that holds as its ideal a loving community:

> The correct understanding of the religion of Jesus inhered in the creation of community, and thus in right living rather than right belief, because love is ultimately recognized in community. God is love, a pattern of life described as mutuality . . . The inalienable connection between love and justice had its source in mutuality. (Legge, *The Grace of Difference*, 43)

This is a Christianity that does not place its hopes in the rewards of an eternal other-worldly order, but in a this-worldly community that envisages Jesus as the model for all who strive to overcome poverty, oppression and all forms of injustice.[25] So the good and flourishing life is one where justice prevails. In her contextualized and pluralist ethics, Legge is sensitive to the multifaceted axes of difference as they divide and unite women. Her quarrel is not with reason, even less with men, but with the ignorance and pride with which reason has been aligned in its demarcations of justice. If ethics is to be concerned with justice, it can no longer simply dictate injunctions in abstract concepts. It must pay attention to the particulars, to the variety and complexity of voices whose situations have, in the past, excluded them from consideration. Ethics cannot remain elite and remote, a weapon of those who manipulate power, it must be responsive and responsible to all.

Conclusion

Just as feminism itself cannot be standardized, the contributions of feminist thought to ethics cannot be condensed into a cohesive set of observations that would be acceptable to all types of feminism. Yet the three varieties I have selected, while not mutually compatible, all propose revisions to the understanding of reason as it has been employed in ethical thinking. An ethics of equality brings to attention the fact that reason has been discriminatory in its applications of rules and rights. Women, in particular their bodies, have been regulated in ways that have denied, and continue to deny, them recognition as full moral agents who are entitled to, and capable of exercising, the same privileges as men. To argue for parity of treatment however, is not to argue for identity. There will always be matters of prime importance to women, such as decisions concerning their bodies, where their autonomy is to be respected. This does not preclude collaborative consideration, but women can no longer be regarded as objects of control by men.

An ethics of difference demonstrates how reason has been engendered so as to allocate certain virtues and values as either masculine or feminine. These divisions have then been applied, somewhat simplistically, to actual men and women, and those associated with women are regarded as inferior. Ethically this has resulted in women being identified with, for example, the private sphere and moral virtues such as compassion, while men, in the public sphere, monopolize the intellectual virtues such as justice and courage. While some feminists argue that the impersonal and a-historical character of masculine ethics needs tempering by the intimate and particular predisposition of the feminine, others question how these loaded descriptions came to have the restrictive influence they do. All indicators point to the social construction of the definition of knowledge, and thus the question becomes one that ponders the Western heritage's attitude to women and those qualities it deems feminine. If the attributes and applications of knowledge are the product of certain historical and cultural preferences, these can be renegotiated. Thus, an ethics of difference introduces the possibility of removing gender bias from the operations of reason and ethics. Care need not be opposed to justice. Men and women can employ both modes.

Finally, an ethics of pluralism indicates how reason can be selective in its urge to universalize. While this undertaking can often have a corrective intention as, for example, to argue for the rights of all women, it can too easily presume to dictate the terms of their representation. Thus, women of color, women from the third world, or women of non-Western cultures, who have not been consulted before such pronouncements, can feel they have been affiliated with positions they do not hold. Such a topic can be extremely sensitive, and debates range from whether the fault lies in the presumed homogeneity of Western reason (which can itself be a stereotype) to whether Western women (again a problematic label) are as exclusive as Western men in their dealings with the other. What seems to be at stake is the notion that the prescriptions of reason, with particular reference to ethics, can decree in an absolute fashion what either is, or should be, the rule.

In an increasingly multi-cultural and pluralist world, rational processes may still be employed to arrive at a consensus—which is itself an intricate and precarious process—but a communal form of mediation is being sought. On a grand scale this may involve a careful reexamination of the presuppositions of rationality that underlie ethics, but at the very least it will put into question the assumed impersonal and combatively individualistic nature of rationality in its modernist manifestation. In various ways, all three forms of ethics presented here undertake a similar task of interrogation.

Notes

1. There is a debate concerning the division of sex (biology) and gender (culture), with the latter's designation of "masculine" and "feminine" characteristics. Nevertheless, it is instructive to read the works of male philosophers for their assumptions in this regard. See Nancy Tuana, *Woman and the History of Philosophy*, 2–8.

2. See Rosemarie Tong, *Feminine & Feminist Ethics*.

3. Margaret Farley, "Feminist Ethics," *The Westminster Dictionary of Christian Ethics*, 229–31; Claudia Card, ed., *Feminist Ethics*; Eve Browning Cole and Susan Coultrap-McQuin, eds., *Explorations in Feminist Ethics*; Elizabeth J. Porter, *Women and Moral Identity*; Debra Shogun ed., *A Reader in Feminist Ethics*; Marsha Hanen and Kai Nielsen, eds., *Science, Morality & Feminist Theory*, supplementary vol. 13, Canadian Journal of Philosophy; Susan Sherwin, "Ethics, 'Feminine' Ethics, and Feminist Ethics," in *A Reader in Feminist Ethics*, ed. D. Shogun, 3–28; Katie G. Cannon, *Black Womanist Ethics*; Barbara Andolsen, Christine Gudorf and Mary Pellauer, eds., *Women's Consciousness, Women's Conscience: A Reader in Feminist Ethics*.

4. As is the custom in much contemporary writing, feminist and otherwise, an author situates her writings with regard to those influences that have been formative. As a white, heterosexual, middle-class, university-employed female, born in Australia, working in Canada, my sympathies have always predisposed me to issues of justice, particularly regarding the displaced and the dispossessed. But having "one's head in the right place," is, I have become aware, not sufficient to counter the systemic and inculcated prejudices that operate at unconscious levels. These can be, and often are, both self-destructive and damaging to others whose backgrounds are at variance with my own. Within feminist ethics there is a growing appreciation that the rhetoric

of justice, though necessary, is not sufficient to change such inequities. This essay explores what other approaches may help alleviate the discriminations of many types that exist in most Western-influenced societies.

5. It is worth noting that it is not just women who have been excluded—it has basically been one class of males that has presided over learning in general. Males of different classes, as well as slaves, colonized peoples, and those of other cultures have also been designated as not conforming to the qualities and properties consistent with Western reason. I would also concede that Western reason is not monolithic and there have been various schools over the centuries. However, in all of them, women are not credited with having rational or ethical capabilities.

6. See Moira Gatens, "Women and Her Double(s): Sex, Gender and Ethics," Chapter 3 in *Imaginary Bodies: Ethics, Power and Corporeality.*

7. For a treatment of Aristotle, see Nancy Tuana, *Woman and the History of Philosophy*, 23–30. For Kant, see Nancy Tuana, *Woman and the History of Philosophy*, 58–70 and Genevieve Lloyd, *The Man of Reason*, 64–70. For Hegel, see Nancy Tuana, *Woman and the History of Philosophy*, 98–108 and Genevieve Lloyd, *The Man of Reason*, 70–3.

8. Sigmund Freud, "Some Psychical Consequences of the Anatomical Distinction Between the Sexes," in *The Standard Edition of the Complete Psychological Works of Freud* 19, ed. J. Strachey, 257–8.

9. For further study see Christine Gudorf, *Body, Sex and Pleasure: Reconstructing Christian Sexual Ethics.*

10. Harrison supports "a consensus favoring the legal availability of safe surgical abortion," at the same time as she holds that "the act of abortion is sometimes, even frequently, a positive moral good for women" (*Our Right to Choose*, 16). Harrison does not attempt to delineate specific policies, as she believes the diversity of women's situations will require particular assessment.

11. In particular, see Harrison's discussion of "body-right," in *Our Right to Choose*, 196–7.

12. See Beverly Harrison, *Our Right to Choose*, 18–27, 196–200, and 231–44.

13. Harrison is uncompromising in her indictment of not just abortion policy, but of the social and economic conditions that make abortion a necessary option of birth control for poor women, while allow the rich the customary consolations of privilege.

14. See Eva Feder Kittay and Diana T. Meyers, eds., *Women and Moral* for a comprehensive debate about Gilligan's work.

15. The term "essentialism" is used to refer to definitions of women that presume there are fixed and intrinsic qualities that belong to all women.

16. Sarah Lucia Hoagland, "Some Thoughts about 'Caring,'" in *Feminist Ethics*, ed. Claudia Card, 236–46 ; Sabina Lovibond, "Maternalist Ethics: A Feminist Assessment," *South Atlantic Quarterly*, vol. 93 no. 4 (1994): 779–802; Review Symposium on Nel Noddings, *Hypatia*, vol. 5 no. 1 (1990): 101–25.

17. Nancy Scheper-Hughes, "Mother Love," *New Internationalist*, no. 254 (1994): 11–14.

18. Joy Kroeger-Mappes, "The Ethic of Care vis-à-vis the Ethic of Rights: A Problem for Contemporary Moral Theory," *Hypatia*, vol 9, no. 3 (1994): 108–31.

19. Kathryn Tanner, "The Care that Does Justice: Recent Writings in Feminist Ethics and Theology," *Journal of Religious Ethics* 24 (1996): 171–91; Elizabeth Ann Bartlett, "Beyond Either/Or: Justice and Care in the Ethics of Albert Camus," in *Explorations in Feminist Ethics*, ed. Eve Browning Cole and Susan Coultrap-McQuin, 82–8; Marilyn Friedman, "Beyond Caring: The De-Moralization of Gender," in *An Ethic of Care*, ed. Mary Jeanne Larrabee, 258–73.

20. Sarah Hoagland, *Lesbian Ethics: Toward a New Value*; Marilyn Frye, "A Response to *Lesbian Ethics*: Why Ethics?" in *Feminist Ethics*, ed. Claudia Card, 52–9.

21. Postmodernism is a notoriously difficult concept to describe. Basically a protest against the smug certainties of modernism, it ranges far and wide in its applications. It has both nihilistic adherents who do not wish to be constrained by what they believe are artificial standards, and more moderate advocates who view it as a form of protest against a-historical generalizations and grand narratives (even feminist ones). For a discussion of the various options as they are played out in feminist theory see: Margaret Ferguson and Jennifer Wicke eds., *Feminism and Postmodernism*.

22. These remarks are made in the context of a discussion of the work of Dolores Williams, "The Color of Feminism," *Journal of Religious Thought* 43, no. 1, (1986): 42–58.

23. The term womanist is used by many African-American women as a term to distinguish them from white feminists. For an excellent overview of their work in ethics, see Cheryl J. Sanders, "Womanist Ethics: Contemporary Trends and Themes," in *Annual of the Society for Christian Ethics*, 299–305. See also, Roundtable Discussion, "Christian Ethics and Theology in Womanist Perspective," *Journal of Feminist Studies in Religion*, vol.5, no. 2, (1989), 83–112.

24. For a comprehensive coverage that witnesses to these voices see Gloria Anzaldúa, ed., *Making Face, Making Soul, Haciendo Caras: Creative and Critical Perspectives by Women of Color*.

25. These are certain of the tenets of liberation theology. See Gustavo Gutiérrez, *A Theology of Liberation: History, Politics, and Salvation*, trans. and ed. Sister Caridad Inda and John Eagleson.

Works Cited

Andolsen, Barbara, Christine Gudorf, and Mary Pellauer, eds. 1985. *Women's Consciousness, Women's Conscience: A Reader in Feminist Ethics*. Minneapolis: Winston Press.

Anzaldúa, Gloria, ed. 1990. *Making Face, Making Soul,* Haciendo Caras: *Creative and Critical Perspectives by Women of Color*. San Francisco: Aunt Lute Foundation Books.

Bartlett, Elizabeth Ann. 1992. "Beyond Either/Or: Justice and Care in the Ethics of Albert Camus." In *Explorations in Feminist Ethics: Theory and Practice*, edited by Eve Browning Cole and Susan Coultrap-McQuin. 82-8. Bloomington, IN: Indiana University Press.

Braidotti, Rosi. 1994. *Nomadic Subjects: Embodiment and Sexual Difference in Contemporary Feminist Theory*. New York: Columbia University Press.

Cannon, Katie G. 1988. *Black Womanist Ethics*. Atlanta: Scholars Press.

Card, Claudia, ed. 1991. *Feminist Ethics*. Lawrence, KS: University Press of Kansas.

Cole, Eve Browning, and Susan Coultrap-McQuin, eds. 1992. *Explorations in Feminist Ethics: Theory and Practice*. Bloomington, IN: Indiana University Press.

Farley, Margaret. 1986 "Feminist Ethics," *The Westminster Dictionary of Christian Ethics*. Philadelphia: The Westminster Press.

Ferguson, Margaret, and Jennifer Wicke, eds. 1994. *Feminism and Postmodernism*. Durham, NC: Duke University Press.

Freud, Sigmund. 1961 "Some Psychical Consequences of the Anatomical Distinction Between the Sexes." In *The Standard Edition of the Complete Psychological Works of Freud* 19, edited by J. Strachey, 248–58. London: Hogarth Press.

Friedman, Marilyn. 1993. "Beyond Caring: The De-Moralization of Gender." In *An Ethic of Care*, edited by Mary Jeanne Larrabee. New York: Routledge.

Frye, Marilyn. 1991. "A Response to *Lesbian Ethics*: Why Ethics?" In *Feminist Ethics*, edited by Claudia Card. Lawrence, KS: University Press of Kansas.

Gatens, Moira. 1996. *Imaginary Bodies: Ethics, Power and Corporeality*. New York: Routledge.

Gilligan, Carol. 1982. *In a Different Voice: Psychological Theory and Women's Development*. Cambridge: Harvard University Press.

Gudorf, Christine. 1994. *Body, Sex and Pleasure: Reconstructing Christian Sexual Ethics*. Cleveland: Pilgrim Press.

Gutiérrez, Gustavo. 1973. *A Theology of Liberation: History, Politics, and Salvation*. Translated and edited by Sr. Caridad Inda and John Eagleson. Maryknoll, NY: Orbis Books.

Hanen, Marsha, and Kai Nielsen, eds. 1987. *Science, Morality & Feminist Theory*. Calgary: University of Calgary Press.

Harrison, Beverly Wildung. 1985. *Making the Connections: Essays in Feminist Social Ethics*. Boston: Beacon Press.

———. 1983. *Our Right to Choose: Toward a New Ethic of Abortion*. Boston: Beacon Press.

Hoagland, Sarah Lucia. 1988. *Lesbian Ethics: Toward New Value*. Palo Alto, CA: Institute of Lesbian Studies.

Kittay, Eva Feder, and Diana T. Meyers, eds. 1987. *Women and Moral Theory*. Totowa, NJ: Rowman & Littlefield.

Kroeger-Mappes, Joy. 1994. "The Ethics of Care vis-à-vis the Ethic of Rights: A Problem for Contemporary Moral Theory." *Hypatia* 9, no 3: 108–131.

Legge, Marilyn J. 1992. *The Grace of Difference: A Canadian Feminist Theological Ethic.* Atlanta: Scholars Press.

Lloyd, Genevieve. 1985. *The Man of Reason: "Male" and "Female" in Western Philosophy.* Minneapolis: University of Minnesota Press.

Lovibond, Sabina. 1994. "Maternalist Ethics: A Feminist Assessment." *South Atlantic Quarterly* 93, no. 4: 779–802.

Lugones, María. 1987. "Playfulness, 'World'-Traveling and Loving Perception." In *Hypatia*, vol. 2, no. 2: 17.

Noddings, Nel. 1984. *Caring: A Feminist Approach to Ethics and Moral Education.* Berkeley: University of California Press.

Porter, Elizabeth J. 1991. *Women and Moral Identity.* Sydney: Allen & Unwin.

Ruddick, Sara. 1989. *Maternal Thinking: Toward a Politics of Peace.* Boston: Beacon Press.

Sanders, Cheryl J. 1989. "Christian Ethics and Theology in Womanist Perspective." In *Journal of Feminist Studies in Religion 5*, no 2: 83–112.

———. 1994. "Womanist Ethics: Contemporary Trends and Themes." In the *Annual of the Society for Christian Ethics.* Washington: Georgetown Press.

Scheper-Hughes, Nancy. 1994. "Mother Love." In *New Internationalist* 254: 11–14.

Sherwin, Susan. 1993. "Ethics, 'Feminine' Ethics, and Feminist Ethics." In *A Reader in Feminist Ethics,* edited by D. Shogun, 39–56. Toronto: Canadian Scholars Press, Inc.

Shogun, Debra, ed. 1993. *A Reader in Feminist Ethics.* Toronto: Canadian Scholars Press, Inc.

Tanner, Kathryn. 1996. "The Care that Does Justice: Recent Writings in Feminist Ethics and Theology." In *Journal of Religious Ethics* 24: 171–191.

Tong, Rosemarie. 1993. *Feminine & Feminist Ethics.* Belmont, CA: Wadsworth Publishers.

Tuana, Nancy. 1992. *Woman and the History of Philosophy.* New York: Paragon House.

Williams, Dolores. 1986. "The Color of Feminism." In *Journal of Religious Thought*, vol. 43, no. 1: 42–58.

Yeatman, Anna. 1994. *Postmodern Revisionings of the Political.* New York: Routledge.

Chapter 10

Are there Religious Responses to Global Ethical Issues?

Harold Coward

Each of us is today faced with the challenge of how we respond to global problems such as population pressure, excess consumption and environmental degradation. Ozone holes, the Greenhouse warming of the atmosphere, pollution of water and destruction of fish and forests are problems caused by human intervention in the processes of nature—processes of which we humans are an interdependent part. Scientists and non-government organizations (NGO's) have done a good job in detailing these problems.[1] Scientists, however, cannot solve these problems for what is required is nothing short of radical changes in behavior. In religious language, a "conversion" in our lifestyle is needed from most Canadians, Americans, Europeans and the well-off classes in developing countries which consume just as excessively as do the well-off in Canada. The issues are ethical—will we and our children make the choices that will leave enough of nature's resources to sustain future children for up to seven generations (to use an Aboriginal rule of thumb)? To change one's behavior and lifestyle is never easy, but it is one area where the religions have something special to offer—for down through the ages it is the religions that have a track record of success in changing people. Even as secular a journal as *The Economist* recognizes this in its December 21, 1966 issue which features an article titled "Godliness and Greenness: Thou shalt not covet the earth," arguing that our environmental problems can only be solved by "an awareness of something higher. . . ."[2] Today, on all sides, religious wisdom for life ethics is being called forth.

These challenges of over population, excess consumption of the world's resources, and the pollution of earth, air, and water are new ethical problems that call forth new theology challenging each tradition to search its teachings for relevant wisdom.

Paul Tillich proposed that theology proceeds by what he called "a correlational method" (Tillich, *Systematic Theology*, 61). In response to the challenges and questions posed by human existence, theology searches its sources of revelation and tradition for answers. It is only recently that the various religions have had to question their sources with regard to the interaction of humans with the environment—in response to the explosion in numbers of people and their consumption of the earth's resources at a rate that threatens to exhaust its life sustaining capacity. Thus the advent of ecotheology in Christianity in which the themes of nature and environment (which one searches for in vain in earlier thinkers) are a "cutting edge" issue of the day (see, for example, Ruether's *Gaia and God*, and McFague's *The Body of God*). It is perhaps not a surprise that much of this ecotheologizing is being done by women scholars, for the analysis suggests that just as nature has often been treated as a resource to be exploited, so have women. Indeed Rosemary Ruether argues that patriarchal societies and religions have categorized women together with nature and treated both as commodities to be used. She says, "what is necessary is a double transformation of both women and men in their relation to each other and to 'nature'"(Ruether, *Gaia and God*, 265). She offers militarism as the strongest example of this double rape of both women and the earth, and concludes that the change of consciousness needed "is one that recognizes that real 'security' lies, not in dominating power and the impossible quest for total invulnerability, but rather in the acceptance of vulnerability, limits, and interdependency with others, with other humans and with the earth" (268). In the Hindu context, Vandana Shiva offers a similar critique.

The ecofeminist theology response points up the necessity of a fresh approach to the population problem. Rather than the imposition of *fertility control* via demographic quotas to be met by the introduction of family planning so as to slow population growth (funded largely by the United States Agency for International Development), the new approach introduced during the lead-up to the Cairo summit is *reproductive health*. It signals a change from seeing the population pressure problem as subject to a scientific solution through the imposition of medical technology (a 'control' approach often through sterilization of the woman) to a holistic approach which involves "reducing poverty, improving health, decreasing mortality rates, enhancing education, augmenting reproductive health services, achieving sustainable development, abating environmental degradation and excessive consumption, and attaining gender equity and equality" (Grist and Greenfield, "Population and Development," 50). The voices of women from NGO's and religions around the world were a powerful influence in achieving this significant shift in approach at Cairo. What it makes clear for theologians of all religions is that one can no longer deal with the challenges of population pressure, excess consumption and environmental degradation as questions to be addressed separately.

While this makes matters more complex, it also opens the door to exciting "new theology." When, following Tillich's correlational method, we ask our traditions for their wisdom on the three-pronged problematic of population, consumption and ecology, we find fresh and creative answers forth-coming—answers that we could not get by asking about the ethics of reproduction, just consumption and our relation to nature separately. I say this on the basis of personal experience. Some years ago I put together an interdisciplinary research team to do an ethical analysis of possible scientific and social responses to the challenge of the greenhouse effect. In analyzing the teachings of the various religions, I was able to sift out their "theologies of nature,"[3] but the result was unsatisfying because it remained at the level of theory and lacked the ability to engage the world's very real problems. A major weakness in the study was our failure to include the population variable. Even if decision-makers in governments and in the private sector made the "green" choice based on our ethical analysis, the environmental threat would continue to worsen due to the increase in the earth's population. As a result, in 1993 under the auspices of the Center for Studies in Religion and Society at the University of Victoria, I brought together a new team of scientists, social scientists, secular philosophers and theologians to re-examine the issue with the population variable included.[4] But scholars from the developing countries—especially from India—quickly convinced us that to look at population without consumption resulted in an unjust "saddling" of the developing countries of the South with both the problem and the responsibility for its solution—because it is in those countries that the rapid population growth of today and in the future decades will take place, yet it is the few babies born in the developed countries that will excessively consume and pollute the environment. Thus we were forced to enlarge our focus from environment and population to include issues of consumption of the earth's resources (sustainability and just sharing). Consequently, our three-pronged problematic. In no religion could we find this complex multifaceted problematic already addressed. The task called for truly new theology from each religion. The result was exciting for although we could only begin the task, new creative openings began to appear. For example, our Muslim scholar found that the *Qur'an* teaches that humans, as custodians of nature, are free to satisfy their own needs *only* with an eye to the welfare of all creation. Thus, humans must share natural resources and population pressure will dictate limits to consumption so that there can be equal access to resources by all. While fertility control is generally forbidden by the *Qur'an*, and the production of children encouraged, the putting together of the Qur'anic teaching on nature and consumption, with reproduction, provides a way of suggesting that fertility control may be acceptable if seen as part of self-discipline required from humans to avoid upsetting the divinely created balance of nature.

In the Jewish tradition the mystical thought of the Kabbalists suggests that humans must learn to limit themselves—their rate of reproduction, their use of natural resources and their production of fouling wastes. As humans we are to pattern our behavior after the example God gives in the creation of the world. If God is omnipresent then, reasoned the Kabbalists, the only way God could create would be by an act of *tsimtsum*—of voluntary withdrawal or limitation to make room for creation. Similarly, we as humans must withdraw or limit both our reproduction and our wants, so as to make room for coexistence with our environment in this and future generations. As one scholar puts it: "The miracle of co-habitation with other living species, the beauty of collective I-Thou relationship with beings wholly different from ourselves, requires our self-limitation. If we were everywhere, our presence would herald the end of the teeming diversity of nature. Our fragile and unique habitat needs a reprieve from Human assault" (Schorsch, "Trees for Life," 6).

A Christian scholar on our research team concluded that Christianity had a major responsibility for fostering much of the world's excessive consumption and overpopulation.[5] Yet within Christianity there are strong forces at work transforming Christianity's mainstream into a self-critical force for justice, peace, and the maintenance of the integrity of nature. The ecology of the planet cannot be separated from population and social justice concerns when seen through Christian feminist theology. In this context, the traditional Christian opposition to fertility control is just beginning to be critically examined in relation to the looming crisis of overpopulation. Christian thinkers are recognizing, however, that it is over consumption by the developed Christian countries of the North that is both polluting the environment and depriving the developing countries of the South of the resources they need. It is the babies of well-off parents of the first-world who pose the largest threat to the ecology—not the babies of the underdeveloped Asians, Africans or Latin Americans. Therefore, it is the child who has the most, the first-world child, that the world can least afford. This leads Catherine Keller to the radical conclusion that well-off Christians should choose to reduce their own populations and resource consumption, so as to make room for the migrating poor. Such an ascetic choice is not seen by Keller as a denial of pleasure, but as a responsible practice of fertility in relation to others and to nature. It also challenges the traditional patriarchal family patterns basic to many Christian cultures. This teaching, Keller maintains, is in line with the teaching of the Hebrew prophets who maintain that humans and nature are required to live together in justice, and with the teaching of Jesus that one must love one's neighbor in need (e.g., as did the Good Samaritan). Christians today are realizing that their neighbor's welfare is strongly affected by the way they treat the environment and by the number of children they produce. The prophets addressed the issue of resource consumption from the vantage point of the poor. The lesson for Christians today, says Keller, is not to multiply the *quantity* of life, but to enhance the *quality* of life through the sharing of nature's abundance. The result is an ethic of interdependence with the rest of creation, which may also mean an ethic of "non-creation" for well-off Christians—for the good of the whole. For the early New Testament Christians, the notion of an immanent end-time (the second coming of Christ) led them to counsel "few possessions and no children." Christians today are hearing a similar counsel, not because the end (the Apocalypse) is coming, but in order to avoid another kind of end—an ecological catastrophe.

Any analysis of reproduction, consumption and ecology practices raises the question as to who is the ethical agent—the decision-maker in the new theology that will result. I have begun the task of exploring the differences between individual and collective self-identities in ethical decision-making related to our three-fold problematic. Most modern Western thought assumes that the ethical agent is the autonomous individual—the "I-Self" as I call it. Traditional cultures, however, tend to give ethical agents a collective identity—a "We-Self"—which extends outward in varying degrees of inclusiveness from family, caste and tribe to an embrace of animals, plants and even inorganic matter—earth, air and water. While all religions stress the importance of going beyond a narrow, selfish I-Self so as to give ethical standing to others, the breadth of the We-Self embraced tends to expand as one moves East and to the Aboriginal traditions. I want to spend the rest of this chapter examining this distinction for "life ethics" and its relevance for the three-pronged problematic of population, consumption and the environment.

Those of us shaped by a modern Western upbringing and cultural context tend to experience our personal identity as created by our choosing of options. This is the modern liberal concept of individuals as choosers. Our identity in a liberal society is a construct of the choices we make or fail to make. We see ourselves first and foremost as consumers or as constructors of options. Our natural, social and economic environments are then for us not givens but potentially manipulable elements in our never ceasing struggle for, what Thomas Hobbes in the *Leviathan* calls, "power after power." This leads us to seek the maximum benefits for our individual selves here and now over against the good of other persons now, or future generations or nature itself. We tend to structure the world so that the individual choices we make in reproductive, economic or environmental situations will bring us maximum benefit. The ethic encouraged is one of self-interest defined in individualistic, utilitarian terms rather than self-interest through identification with the larger whole; e.g., humanity or the cosmos. It produces a focus upon human rights (often defined as isolated individual rights in law and public policy) as a way of ensuring that each person gets his or her fair share. It fosters an economy which, when meshed with modern technology, constantly expands to supply enlarging needs (with increasing levels of consumption) and to keep pace with the world's rapidly growing population. The result is an unsustainable degradation of nature in the name of serving human needs defined as human rights. Human beings, and their needs, are put at war with the sustainability of nature—which according to some readings of the Bible and Qur'an is created for the purpose of supporting humans. This one-sided ontology may have helped foster the modern liberal emphasis on the individual. When put together with utilitarian secular ethics and the market economy, the results for the global ecosystem may be devastating (see The Greenhouse Effect projections of environmental scientists).[6]

Although the individual as atomistic, isolated chooser is the identity that dominates the self-understanding of most modern Europeans and North Americans, for much of the rest of the world identity is understood quite differently. In traditional Jewish, Islamic, Hindu, Buddhist, Chinese and Aboriginal societies self-identity is constructed not by individual choices but by participating in a "family" which may extend out to include caste, tribe, and all humans as well as plants, animals and the cosmos. For example, in the Chinese world view it is never the isolated, individual "self" but the self as interrelated in community, nature and with heaven that is the ethical agent. Identity is in one's harmonious interrelationships, not in one's choices/rights, powers and privileges. Such a broadened self-understanding leads to a focus on obligations to the whole rather than an emphasis on individual human rights—although the safeguards of the latter are an important defense against abuses of the individual (especially children and women) that the former has sometimes produced, and therefore they need to be retained but balanced. Let me move from the level of broad social, political and economic analysis to that of psychological processes to further explore the different understandings of the self as an ethical agent that I have sketched above. I begin with a personal illustration.

Several years ago when I was just beginning my career as a university professor, I ended up going to a conference with a colleague who was Hindu, born in India. I am a Canadian Protestant Christian. Now I knew all about Hinduism—in fact I taught it in the university. But until this trip I had not really understood the tradition from within. The difference began when we selected our seats on the plane. Of course, we would sit together, but the seats should be chosen so as to avoid certain inauspicious numbers. When we got to the hotel room which we were sharing, other things began to happen. I noticed my friend using my toothpaste. For me, this seemed to be an invasion of my privacy and property, without even the courtesy of asking permission. For him, there was no clear separation of ownership because we were together—our identities and possessions were merged into a collective unity. It was our toothpaste, and as it looked interesting, he was trying it. I soon came to understand that being together also meant that whenever we left the room to attend sessions, eat or do some sightseeing, we did it together. This was quite different from my usual conference-going experience of room sharing where the only time you might see your roommate was at night or on waking in the morning. Being with my Hindu colleague and sharing his world view meant we did everything together. The two of us were merged into one. For me to go off to do something on my own would have caused a serious rupture in our collective personhood. No longer was I an autonomous individual. We made our decisions as a shared identity.

This collective as opposed to individual identity has important implications for issues of population, consumption, and ecology. As doctors, nurses or ethicists dealing with reproductive issues, for example, it means we are not interacting with an autonomous person (our usual experience), but with a person who understands his/her self-identity in terms of a larger whole such as an extended family.

Alan Roland, a New York psychiatrist reports just such an experience.[7] He found that his Indian Hindu patients (highly educated professionals) did not respond to his usual modern Western therapies, which assumed a strongly individualized sense of self—an I-ness characterized by a self-contained set of ego boundaries with sharp distinctions between self and others. By contrast he found his South Asian patients to be a familial or "We-Self" that enabled them to function within extended families. Rather than the self-contained ego boundaries of the typical North American "I-Self" which allows us to function in a highly autonomous society, the "We-Self" of his Indian patients had highly permeable ego boundaries opening the way for the constant empathy and receptivity to others necessary for life in an extended family. Instead of actualization of the individual self, the personal and spiritual goal of the South Asian is the reciprocal responsibility required to live in harmony within the hierarchical structure of family, society and ideally all of nature. Whereas the North American "I-Self" sharply separates between self and others, self and nature, often in a competitive fashion, the We-Self of Asian cultures extends outward to include family, caste-group, linguistic-ethnic culture and even the natural environment. From the Buddhist perspective, which is dominant in the cultures of East and South-East Asia, it is our false attachment to the I-Self and its selfish desires that is the cause of unethical action and suffering. Understanding ourselves as but a tiny interdependent part of the complex "We-Self" of the cosmos leads to compassionate action and *Nirvana*. Yet within that complex "We-Self," observes Roland, a highly private ego is maintained.

What does all this mean for reproductive issues in health care? First, diagnosis and treatment in many cultures will have to pay more attention to the extended family and the environmental context in which the person lives—the "We-Self." For example, my wife, a nurse, working in a family practice unit serving prairie Stony Aboriginal patients had frequent "We-Self" experiences. When a young woman or older teenage girl would arrive with gynaecological problems, she would be accompanied by her mother, aunts and grandmother. All would insist on going back to the examining room together (a room designed to hold just two or three). When the doctor was taking the history, often it would be the grandmother who would do the talking, saying when the girl had had her last period, for example. Everyone knew everything, naturally, as they were a "We-Self." And everyone expected to be involved in the treatment and any ethical decisions to be made. This raises the second point, namely that issues of consent have to take seriously that the ethical decision-maker in such a culture is not just the individual, but the "We-Self" of which they are but a respected part. Recognition of this fact should cause us to re-examine our methods and forms for obtaining consent which, for the most part, are devised on the assumption that the person is an autonomous individual—an I-Self, sharply separated from others in one's family or society. The existence of cultures with "We-Self" expanding identities challenges autonomous conceptions of health and human rights often assumed in United Nations declarations, especially relating to women and children. We should not be surprised to discover that the feminist movements in traditional cultures do not always express the goal for women in terms of individual women's rights. Rather it is the just and respected place of women within the "We-Self" of the family and even the environment that is the focus of ethical analysis. When ethical issues surrounding reproduction arise, a woman within the "We-Self" ideally ponders the good of the extended family and the sustainable capacities of the environment, along with her own desires, in coming to a decision. Nor should we be surprised to find that in such cultures the idea that children or adolescents have ethical standing independent of the family raises reactions of incomprehensibility and hostility.

While our modern Western notions of individual autonomy and human rights can serve to highlight ethical abuses and exploitation that can and do arise in the extended family (an important contribution often liberating to women and children), the other side of the coin is that the "We-Self" ideals of mutual responsibility and respect between ourselves, others and the environment are a much needed corrective to a self-centered selfishness that our modern Western competitive "I-Self" so successfully generates. Indeed at a time of rapid population increase and/or tightened resources in health care, ethical questions as to who gets treatment and in what order of priority are made very difficult, if not impossible to resolve, when the rights of individual autonomy reign supreme. A collective "We-Self," by contrast, provides a more practical and helpful ethical approach, one which strives to balance the needs of the individual with those of the larger interdependent whole. In our current and future scarce resources scenarios, we may find wisdom in the way traditional "We-Self" cultures have developed ethical guidelines for solving such problems. Inuit grandparents used to go off to freeze to death in the snow when there was not enough food for the young. While our technological capacities should enable us to avoid the prescription of freezing to death, the ethical value of the "We-Self" in giving priority to the young in times of scarce resources is one we should carefully consider.

The experience of death in different cultures offers another illustration as to how great sensitivity is demanded in understandings of self-identity. Our autonomous "I-Self" focus has led us to give great attention to such things as advance directives or living wills. This is in sharp contrast to "We-Self" societies where it is inconceivable to think of the death of an individual independent from the community of which he or she is a part. Of course, individuals must have the right to some definite say about their own dying place, even in communitarian societies.

Peter Stephenson, a medical anthropologist, offers an example from a Hutterite community in southern Alberta. In contrast to the fast (and therefore supposedly 'painless') 'ideal death' of an individual in modern Western culture, the Hutterite ideal of a good death is one that is slow and drawn out surrounded by family and community. Everyone is anxious to see the "fortunate one" who is preparing to enter a better heavenly life. Death-bed time is needed for the dying Hutterite for it is a time when, together with the members of their community, "they are to 'relive' their lives, to forgive others and to be forgiven" (Stephenson, "'He Died too Quick!'", 129). Dying is not an isolated matter for the individual self but an obligation to be lived through with the We-Self of the whole community—allowing for the socialization of all into the prospect of a better heavenly life.

How does all of this become an ethical issue for doctors, nurses, and communities? Stephenson tells the story of his Hutterite friend, Paul, who at forty-eight died of lymphosarcoma. Paul was taken from his home colony to hospital in the city. Because of limited visiting hours and distant travel, few members of the community were able to visit Paul and together with him prepare for a good death. Finally after nearly two weeks, Paul was returned to his colony by ambulance arriving in the evening but dying at 4:00 a.m. In the eyes of the community, Paul's death was "too quick." Paul's isolated time in hospital represented a lost opportunity for the collective self of Paul and his community to prepare a good death. Stephenson concludes: "When Paul died he was still too much alive—he was still among the [living] and not yet with 'the dead'"(Stephenson, 132). He did not have time to put his We-Self to rest.

Having described the distinction between the I-Self and We-Self in ethical analysis, let us now carefully examine the relationship between the We-Self and engagement of the individual in ethical action—as for example in responding to the challenges of overpopulation, excess consumption and degradation of the environment. Does understanding oneself as a We-Self rather than I-Self make any difference to the way one responds to these ethical challenges?

Each of us seems to react in an unselfish spontaneous way in sudden situations as, for example, when we come upon an accident on the highway. Seeing the car in the ditch, our immediate impulse is to stop and help—the foot comes off the accelerator and onto the brake. But then in a flash of thought, our "I-Self" mind goes to work: am I really the right person to help, since I am not a doctor or nurse I might not do the right thing and might be sued, therefore, better leave it for someone else more qualified and, besides, if I stop I will be late for my important appointment—and so the foot goes back on to the accelerator. In the extraordinary or perfected person, by contrast, the shadow of selfish thought never darkens the immediate compassionate impulse, the car is braked to a full stop and help given. The injured person is part of one's larger We-Self identity and caring action comes spontaneously, just as it did in Jesus' parable of the Good Samaritan. While the Western religions of Judaism, Christianity and Islam clearly require the extension of our We-Self identities to include all other humans—women, children, the foreigner, and even our enemy—Asian and Aboriginal teaching pushes further until all animals, as well as organic and inorganic nature, are included. Such an all-inclusive We-Self is, I think, potentially present in each of us. We do seem to impulsively pull back from hurting animals, killing plants or polluting earth, air and water. But this momentary We-Self impulse rapidly disappears under the stronger self-interest of the I-Self. Even when our thinking adopts ideals that value social and economic justice along with respect for animals, plants, earth, air and water, our actions do not always follow suit. A mind-body split remains.

For the Western religions, the way to overcome this barrier to compassionate action is through the surrender of one's I-Self to God in obedience. When focused on social justice issues this approach has produced some fine theology (e.g., Reinhold Niebuhr's *The Nature and Destiny of Man*) and some exemplary action including: the Quakers' emancipation of women, opposition to slavery, prison reform and the extension of education to all classes of society; the Mennonites' willingness to fight hunger, poverty and to work for peace; and Martin Luther King Jr.'s movement to liberate blacks in the United States. Until recently, however, Western religious examples of the unification of mind and body into compassionate action that transcends the I-Self seem restricted to the human realm. Only in Western mystical thought (e.g., the Kabbalists of Judaism and the Sufis of Islam or saints like Francis of Assisi) do we find a strong impulse to extend the We-Self beyond humans to identification with animals, plants and the whole of the cosmos. Today it is no longer just the esoteric witness of the mystics that is pushing the extension of the We-Self to include all of nature. It is the challenges of overpopulation, unsustainable consumption and the threatened destruction of the natural ecosystem itself that is forcing Jews, Christians, and Muslims toward an extended We-Self of the sort earlier mystics pioneered.

While the Asian approaches of Hinduism, Buddhism, Chinese Religion and the Aboriginal traditions have all advocated an extended We-Self (inclusive of animals, plants, earth, air and water) from the start,[8] the degree to which this has resulted in more enlightened action in these societies seems open to question. Callicot and Ames have suggested that the differences among religions do not seem to make much difference when we examine how humans have interacted with nature to date. In both the East and the West the environment has been ruthlessly exploited. In the view of Callicot and Ames it is our innate aggressiveness as *Homo sapiens*, inherited from prehuman savanna primates, that is at the root of the problem (Callicot & Ames, "Epilogue," 281). This might lead us to the pessimistic conclusion that what religions teach about ecology does not matter after all, for we as humans are simply driven by our biological inheritance strongly manifested in our modern Western I-Selves. However, neither the religions discussed nor secular ethics would accept such a deterministic position. There is simply too much evidence that humans can and do change their behavior—sometimes in radical fashion. And it is with regard to just such conversions of thought and action that religions have demonstrated success down through the ages.

The particular claim of the Asian traditions is that the perfected realization of the extended We-Self in action is seen as a possibility that everyone of us can achieve—indeed, in Hinduism and Buddhism we will each be reborn as many times as needed until we realize perfection by practicing what we preach. In addition, not only do these religions teach the ideas that each person is perfectible in the fully extended We-Self but they also offer teachers and disciplines (Yoga or meditation techniques) by which we may transform our I-Self behavior into We-Self behavior and so fully unify mind and body in harmony with the cosmos. In more psychological terminology this result would be a unification of the two levels, our ordinary conscious awareness and our unconscious including our neurophysiological body, into a single mind-body unity—a We-Self that is fully aware of the ecosystem of which it is but an interdependent part, and integrated with it in spontaneous ethical action.

Earlier in this chapter, we contrasted the I-Self typical of modern European and North American society with the We-Self that characterizes traditional Muslim, Hindu, Buddhist, Chinese and Aboriginal cultures. It is evident that in these traditional cultures, the We-Self of the vast majority of persons would fall far short of the fully expanded and realized We-Self described in the paragraphs above. In Chinese thought, for example, Mencius[9] distinguishes between the actual and the ideal "We-Self." The question then needs to be raised as to what difference there is between the average actual We-Self in a traditional Hindu, Buddhist, Chinese, Muslim or Aboriginal society and the typical modern European or North American I-Self—especially with regard to ethical action relating to the population, consumption, ecology problematic. The ideal We-Self in traditional cultures made ethical decisions not from an individualistic I-Self perspective but with reference to the larger collective We-Self of which the individual was but a part. With regard to reproduction decisions this means that it is not just the wishes of the woman or the husband and wife that must be considered. The We-Self invokes the extended family and, at times, as in contemporary China, the carrying capacity of the city or country in the action decision (Paper & Paper, "Chinese Religions"). From a Buddhist perspective, concern that population growth may exceed the capacity of the earth may lead to a We-Self decision to moderate both reproduction and consumption (Gross, "Buddhist Resources"). If the We-Self in these traditions takes ethical concern for others no further than the extended family, caste, tribe, or nation, then limiting consumption and making it more just for all people on earth may not happen. Indeed the extended family can be just as powerful a force for greed and environmental exploitation as the individual I-Self. Even within the extended family there can be negative results from We-Self identity—women can be oppressed and led to adopt unhealthy "martyr" roles and children can be looked upon as "pawns" to be moved around for the enhancement of family power and fortune. In Japan, for example, We-Self identification incorporated in industrialism has been most destructive both within and outside of the country in terms of social equity and environmental sustainability. The company functions as a quasi-family providing cradle to grave social security but in turn requiring unquestioning dedication, loyalty and self-sacrifice from its employees. Individual employees may regret spending so little time at home with the family or feel guilt over participation in industrial practices that damage the environment, but the We-Self consciousness that the company has carefully nourished overrides the I-Self conscience of the person as a responsible husband, father, and citizen. Similar destructive We-Self identifications are seen in some "guru-led" organizations like the Om Sinrikyo cult which allegedly sprinkled poisonous gas in the Tokyo subway system. These are the authoritarian or totalitarian We-Self dangers that need an I-Self sense of individual rights and critical conscience so as to maintain a healthy balance. The potential advantage of the person in the extended family is that (as Roland's research demonstrates) from the beginning identity is experienced in a We-Self rather than I-Self form. The lack of individualized ego in the We-Self personality may well make it easier to extend the already existing We-Self personality structure to include justice for all humans and respect for animals, plants, earth, air and water. An added advantage is that many of these We-Self traditions have a fully expanded We-Self identity as the built-in religious goal to be realized—along with the practical techniques for doing it. But what they sometimes lack is the parallel goal of individual critical self-consciousness that is necessary for the development of a non-authoritarian We-Self. Such a We-Self might be characterized as having "unity within diversity"—a person with sufficient individuality as to be able to develop a critical evaluation of those in power and yet retain a sense of being connected to others and to nature leading to compassionate, spontaneous action. This contrasts with the We-Self of a totalitarian kind which is characterized as "unity without diversity." To the outside world, this We-Self can show aggressiveness and chauvinistic denial—as the Japanese examples demonstrate.

To conclude, let us briefly review. We have analyzed the We-Self in relation to its ability to produce ethical action on the issues of population, consumption and ecology. Does being a We-Self rather than an I-Self bring any advantage in this regard? We demonstrated that the non-authoritarian We-Self identity, especially in its Asian or Aboriginal manifestations, opens the way to a more complete realization of ethical action on population, consumption, and ecology than the modern Western I-Self identity offers. Not only is a fully unified mind-body We-Self provided, but in its religious ideal it is extended to include all humans, animals, plants, earth, air and water as the harmonious whole of which the individual is an interdependent part. Further, this ideal is fully realizable in that the ordinary everyday "We-Self" (which may begin by including only the extended family) is expandable via the disciplines of meditation to include all of the cosmos. The practical effect of an expanded and realized We-Self is that in our ethical choosing we are spontaneously restrained, just and compassionate in all matters of reproduction, consumption and ecology. However, this is an ideal that the average We-Self in a traditional Hindu or Buddhist society may take many, many lifetimes to perfect. The We-Self does, however, offer the comparative advantage over the modern Western I-Self of already being a collective identity that by cultivation through spiritual discipline is expandable beyond the family, city or country to identity with the cosmos. In Judaism, Christianity or Islam, this Eastern ideal We-Self is paralleled by the saint or mystic.[10] In all religions, therefore, we find a We-Self ideal which when actualized results in life ethics that would sustain ourselves, future generations, animals, plants, and our natural environment of earth, air and water.

Notes

1. See, for example, T. Houghton, B. A. Callander, and S. K. Varney, eds., *Climate Change: The IPCC Scientific Assessment*; Charles Mann, "How Many Is Too Many?" *Atlantic Monthly*, Feb. 1993; and David Korten, "Sustainability and the Global Economy," in *Visions of a New Earth: Population, Consumption, and Ecology*, ed. Harold Coward and Dan Maguire.

2. "Godliness and Greenness: Thou shalt not covet the earth," *The Economist*, (December 21, 1996), 110.

3. Harold Coward and Thomas Hurka, ed., *Ethics and Climate Change: The Greenhouse Effect*.

4. Harold Coward, ed., *Population, Consumption and the Environment*.

5. Catherine Keller, "A Christian Response to the Population Apocalypse," in *Population, Consumption and the Environment*, 109–22.

6. See Kenneth Hare, "The Natural Background," in *Population, Consumption and the Environment*, chapter 1.

7. Alan Roland, *In Search of Self in India and Japan*.

8. Harold Coward and Thomas Hurka, "Religious Responsibility," in *Ethics and Climate Change: The Greenhouse Effect*, 48–59.

9. Mencius (born about 371 BCE) was a Chinese philosopher and follower of Confucius. He has long been considered the second Sage (to Confucius) by the Chinese.

10. See, for example, the expanded We-Self ideal that Matthew Fox finds in Meister Eckhart, *Breakthrough: Meister Eckhart's Creation Spirituality in New Translation*, Introduction and Commentaries by Matthew Fox, 505.

Works Cited

Callicot, J. B., and R. T. Ames. 1989. "Epilogue: On the Relation of Idea and Action." In *Nature in Asian Traditions of Thought*, edited by J. B. Callicot and R. T. Ames. Albany, NY: State University of New York Press.

Coward, Harold, ed. 1995. *Population, Consumption and the Environment: Religious and Secular Responses*. Albany: State University of New York Press.

Coward, Harold, and Thomas Hurka, eds. 1993. *Ethics and Climate Change: The Greenhouse Effect*. Waterloo, ON: Wilfred Laurier University Press.

Coward, Harold, and Dan Maguire. 1997. *Visions of a New Earth: Population, Consumption, and Ecology*. Albany: State University of New York Press.

Eckhart, Meister. 1980. *Breakthrough: Meister Eckhart's Creation Spirituality in New Translation*. Introduction and commentaries by Matthew Fox. New York: Doubleday.

Grist, A. L. and L. L. Greenfield. 1995. "Population and Development: Conflict and Consensus at Cairo." *Second Opinion* 20, no 4: 41–52.

Gross, Rita, M. 1995. "Buddhist Resources for Issues of Population, Consumption and the Environment." In *Population, Consumption and the Environment: Religious and Secular Responses*. Albany: State University of New York Press, 155–72.

Hare, Kenneth. 1995. "The Natural Background." In *Population, Consumption and the Environment* edited by Harold Coward. Albany: State University of New York Press.

Hobbes, Thomas. *Leviathan*. New York: Liberal Arts Press.

Houghton, J. T., B. A. Callander, and S. K. Varney, eds. 1992. *Climate Change: The IPCC Scientific Assessment*. Cambridge: Cambridge University Press.

Keller, Catherine. 1995. "A Christian Response to the Population Apocalypse." In *Population, Consumption and the Environment* edited by Harold Coward. 109–22.

Mann, Charles. 1993. "How Many Is Too Many?" *Atlantic Monthly*, Feb., vol. 271 issue 2.

McFague, Sallie. 1993. *The Body of God: An Ecological Theology*. Minneapolis: Fortress Press.

Niebuhr, Reinhold. 1964. *The Nature and Destiny of Man: A Christian Interpretation*. Vols 1 and 2. New York: Charles Scribner's Sons.

Paper, Jordan, and Ri Chuang Paper. 1995. "Chinese Religions, Population and the Environment." In *Population, Consumption and the Environment: Religious and Secular Responses*, edited by Harold Coward. Albany: State University of New York Press, 173–91.

Roland, Alan. 1988. *In Search of Self in India and Japan*. Princeton: Princeton University Press.

Ruether, Rosemary Radford. 1992. *Gaia and God: An Ecofeminist Theology of Earth Healing*. San Francisco: Harper.

Schorsch, I. 1992. "Trees for Life." *Melton Journal* 25: 6.

Shiva, Vandana. 1989. Staying Alive: Women, Ecology & Development. London: Zed Books Ltd.

Stephenson, Peter. 1983-1984. "'He Died Too Quick!' The Process of Dying in a Hutterite Colony." *Omega* 14, no. 2, 127–134.

Tillich, Paul. 1951. *Systematic Theology: Reason and Revelation*. Vol 1. Chicago: University of Chicago Press.

List of Contributors

Katharine Bitney is a doctoral student in Religion at the University of Manitoba. Her research area is the Hindu Goddess tradition (Shaktism) and its suitability as a theological framework to Ecofeminism. Her most recent publication is *Singing Bone* (Montréal, The Muses' Company, 1997), a collection of poems.

Harold Coward is Professor of History, and Director of the Center for Studies in Religion and Society at the University of Victoria. His current research includes comparative ethics in the field of environment and health care, and the South Asian Diaspora in Canada. His recent publications include: *Derrida and Indian Philosophy* (SUNY, 1990); *Population, Consumption, and the Environment* (edited, SUNY, 1995), and *Life After Death in World Religions* (edited, Orbis, 1997).

David G. Creamer is a Jesuit priest teaching in the Faculty of Education and Department of Religion at St. Paul's College, University of Manitoba. His research interests include moral and religious education and psychology of religion. A recent book, *Guides for the Journey: John Macmurray, Bernard Lonergan, James Fowler* (University Press of America, 1996), explores congruences in the thought of three significant twentieth-century thinkers.

Laara Fitznor is Metis-Cree, originally from Northern Manitoba. She is Assistant Professor, Faculty of Education, University of Manitoba. She teaches Cross Cultural/Anti-Racism and Aboriginal education to university students. She is currently working on her Doctorate of Education at Toronto's Ontario Institute for Studies in Education. Her thesis topic is "Understanding Aboriginal Educators' Experiences Working Within a Eurocentric Educational System."

Morny Joy, Professor in the Department of Religious Studies at the University of Calgary, has published many articles on women and religion, feminist theory and continental philosophy. She is Past-President of the Canadian Society for the Study of Religion. Her recent publications include two edited books, *Gender, Genre and Religion* (Wilfrid Laurier Press, 1995) and *Paul Ricoeur and Narrative* (University of Calgary Press, 1997).

Klaus K. Klostermaier is Distinguished Professor, Department of Religion, University of Manitoba. He has published extensively on Hinduism, science and religion, hermeneutics and inter-religious dialogue. His many books include *A Survey of Hinduism* (SUNY, 1989) and *Mythologies and Philosophies of Salvation in the Theistic Traditions of the West* (Wilfrid Laurier University Press, 1984).

Dawne C. McCance, Professor and Head, Department of Religion, University of Manitoba, teaches and publishes in the areas of ethics, body history, hermeneutics and continental philosophy. Her recent publications include the book *Posts: Re Addressing the Ethical* (SUNY, 1996).

Sheila McDonough, originally from Calgary, Alberta, teaches courses in World Religions, Islam, and Women and Religion at Concordia University in Montréal. Her publications include *Muslim Ethics and Modernity* (Wilfrid Laurier University Press, 1984) and *Gandhi's Response to Islam* (D. K. Printworld, 1994).

Eva K. Neumaier teaches Tibetan and Buddhist studies at the University of Alberta. Her areas of specialization comprise the literature of *rDzogs-chen* (Great Perfection), the interpretation of sacred biographies, and the interaction between culture in general and literary Buddhism. She has extensively published in academic journals and authored or co-authored several books, of which the most recent is *The Sovereign All-Creating Mind—The Motherly Buddha*, a translation of the *Kun-byed rgyal-po'i mdo* (1992).

Neal Rose, a Jewish Rabbi, is Associate Professor, Department of Religion, University of Manitoba. His interests include religion and healing and story-telling. His most recent publication is an essay on his own spiritual journey, "Fragments of Hasidic Spirituality," in *The Fifty-Eighth Century* (Jason Aaronson Inc., 1996).

Albert Welter is Associate Professor of Religious Studies, University of Winnipeg. His research focus is Chinese Buddhism. His recent publications include *The Meaning of Myriad Good Deeds: A Study of Yung-ming Yen-shou and the Wan-shan t'ung-kuei chi* (Peter Lang, 1993) and a forthcoming article, "A Buddhist Response to the Confucian Revival: Tsan-ning and the Debate over Chinese Culture (Wen) in the Early Sung," in *Sung Buddhism*, eds. Daniel A. Getz and Peter N. Gregory (University of Hawaii).

Index

Note: "n" refers to Notes
        "w" refers to Works Cited